FROM CLASSROOM TO CLINICIAN

HOW TO PRACTICE MEDICINE SAFELY AND CONFIDENTLY AS A NEW GRADUATE NURSE PRACTITIONER OR PHYSICIAN ASSISTANT

JOHN STANGL, PA-C

TABLE OF CONTENTS

INTRODUCTION

"Being a new grad sucks. There, I said it. I knew it wouldn't be easy, but WOW this first job out of school has me questioning if I'm cut out to be a provider. I'm not confident and imposter syndrome is getting to me. Sometimes I wonder, what the heck did I even learn during my years in PA school? There is a ton that I have no idea how to handle. And even for the things I know, I'm not confident enough to make a decision. *What is wrong with me?*"

ANONYMOUS NEW GRAD PA-C

Sound familiar? I have heard stories like this every month for as long as I can remember. The stress and anxiety are palpable. I felt the same way at my first job and so does every new graduate, whether they admit it or not.

Transitioning to practice is an immense challenge for us as advanced practice providers (APPs). There is a knowledge gap between where we are left after graduation and where we need to be for medical practice.

We have historically relied on employers to bridge the gap. However, practices are under increasing stress as patient volumes increase and reimbursements decrease. Employer support for new graduates is stretched thin. APP residency programs remain a great option, but many cannot choose this option for financial or logistical reasons.

That leaves each of us struggling to bridge the gap ourselves. Yet, navigating this journey without mentorship can be inefficient and overwhelming. What's more, it takes several years to learn clinical medicine. **How can new graduates deliver care safely in the interim?**

This is the new grad guidebook, and it will share clear guidance on overcoming this central challenge in your new career. You will learn how to:

- Find a **"safety net job"** with mentorship and oversight.
- Overcome **counter-productive emotions** like imposter syndrome.
- Ramp up quickly to the **practical duties** of your job.
- Use **order sets** responsibly for your specialty's most common presentations.
- Leverage **"external brains"** to help you order and interpret tests correctly.
- Level up your **clinical evaluation skills** with specific techniques to avoid misdiagnosis.
- Prescribe **medications** safely and effectively.
- **Communicate and document well** in patient presentations, consultations, and admissions.
- Identify any patient's **risk of bad outcomes**, so you know when to ask for help.
- Understand and overcome the common **cognitive errors** new graduates make.
- Implement the **risk-mitigation best practices**.

WHO AM I?

I am a practicing PA and clinical educator with nearly a decade of experience. I attended Einstein Medical Center's 18-month emergency medicine PA residency program along with a class of physician residents. I saw first-hand how new physicians are trained and understand why it is the gold standard.

Since then, I have worked in high-acuity emergency medicine and am now an assistant program director at the Washington Emergency Care Physicians APP post-graduate training program. Helping new grads get up to speed is my job now, and I love what I do.

I have walked the path of the stressed and overwhelmed new clinician. Those old emotions resurface when I hear about others' struggles. I wrote this book to address these challenges and make this transition smoother for all.

THE BOOK'S FOCUS

I recognize the new grad reality — you can't learn everything immediately. The book's content will narrow your focus in three ways.

First, it details the *subset of clinical medicine* needed to keep you and your patients safe. Namely, how to detect high-risk conditions and avoid causing iatrogenic harm. With these skills, you'll know when to seek help immediately and when you have time to sort things out.

Second, it narrows your focus to the *subset of patients* you are most likely to miss things: the mid-acuity patient. Healthy patients with mild complaints are low-risk, and critically ill patients are easy to spot. The patients in the middle are the most challenging. These patients look well but have comorbidities or subtle clues for danger that we must recognize.

Lastly, the book highlights the *most common mistakes* new graduates are prone to making, so you know how to avoid them. Each chapter includes these clinical pearls and pitfalls.

To accomplish these goals, you'll need to learn a combination of soft and hard skills. The first few sections discuss soft skills, like how to make great first impressions with your new coworkers and find a mentor. Most of the book then dives into hard skills and fundamental medical knowledge, like pattern recognition for dangerous lab abnormalities.

The target audience for this book is new graduate APPs who will assess, diagnose, and treat patients with medical complaints. The content is relevant for most specialties. This book seeks to reinforce the essential foundations of general medicine before you delve too far into a specialty-specific focus. However, surgicalists and outpatient practices managing previously diagnosed chronic diseases may not benefit.

———

This book will not replace your schooling, on-the-job training, or comprehensive specialty textbooks. Instead, it will give you a sneak peek into your future life and summarize the key knowledge you'll need to succeed.

Your journey will be challenging, but it is worth it. On the other end awaits a gratifying career. I hope you think of me as your mentor and friend, cheering you on each step of the way.

Let's begin!

PART ONE
THE NEXT PHASE

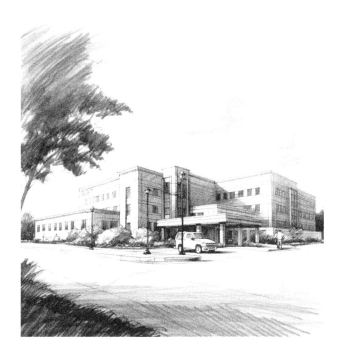

CHAPTER 1
NORMALIZING NEW GRAD EMOTIONS

"I'm in my last year of NP school at a top brick-and-mortar institution and will graduate soon. I'm currently doing my internal medicine rotation, and I am completely overwhelmed at how little I know! The residents and APPs discuss patient cases and I struggle to keep up.

I want to be a knowledgeable NP who can carry myself on a team, but I feel so far behind. Imposter syndrome sucks. When does this get better?"

GRADUATING NP STUDENT, 2022

GRADUATING from a PA or NP program is a tremendous achievement. As you transition into clinical practice, it's natural to encounter a whirlwind of emotions. Some of these emotions will be positive, but many will be negative.

While negative feelings are common, they can quickly become counterproductive if not managed effectively. Excessive stress and anxiety can impair your learning in this important year that demands rapid growth.

Emotions are your first hurdle to overcome in the next phase. This chapter focuses on the most common new graduate experiences and the strategies to overcome them:

- Embarrassment

- Low Confidence
- Imposter Syndrome
- Mindset Challenges
- Motivation Challenges
- Balancing Work and Personal Life

MOVE PAST EMBARRASSMENT

In my first week rounding with a large team in the hospital, an attending told me, "John, get a hold of the disaster lab for this patient." I thought to myself, *That's bizarre — I've never heard of anything like that before. But this patient is very sick and I'm too nervous to ask...*

I got on the phone in front of everyone and asked the hospital operator for the "Disaster lab, please." The whole group burst out laughing, and my attending said, "You misheard—I asked for the vascular lab!" My face turned beet red, and I wanted to hide in a closet.

My coworker put his arm around my shoulder with a smile and said, "Don't worry about it. We all make mistakes like this at first. Don't take things too seriously!" I shrugged off the embarrassment and accepted the hilarity of the situation.

I realize now moments like these help us jumpstart relationships with our coworkers. Even now, years later, the occasional sick patient will prompt a smiling coworker to ask me for a STAT call to the infamous disaster lab.

The takeaway: Mistakes are inevitable, and most will be inconsequential. Instead of stressing over them, try to **laugh it off and move on**. Some mistakes will be quite funny!

UNDERSTAND AND ACCEPT LOW CONFIDENCE

I remember feeling jealous of one classmate who boasted supreme confidence at graduation and "hit the ground running" in their first job. Meanwhile, I felt as if I didn't know anything.

Years later, my mentor taught me about the Dunning-Kruger effect and shared a valuable lesson: low confidence is a *good* sign. It reflects your insight into the immense challenge that is practicing medicine. Those with unfounded faith in their abilities are the most dangerous of all. The ideal mindset for the new graduate is a humble acknowledgment of your clinical limitations paired with enthusiasm and determination to grow.

A similar emotion is *imposter syndrome*, the feeling that you don't truly belong. It's as if you've somehow sneaked in the back door, and it's only a matter of time before you are kicked out.

Whether your classmates admit it or not, we all feel this way initially. The truth is we do deserve to be here. Before long, every one of us becomes a competent clinician and benefits our communities.

The takeaway: Accept that you have low confidence for now. **Develop a plan** to reach competence that you are happy with. Then, put one foot in front of the other and **trust the process**. With each passing month, your confidence will naturally grow.

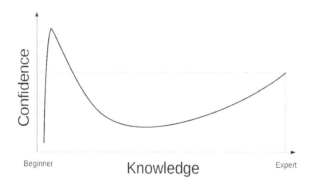

Dunning-Kruger Effect: The least competent people are prone to overestimate their abilities and have a false sense of confidence. They are in a state of "unconscious incompetence." Figure by Jens Egholm Pedersen, with permission.

ADOPT A GROWTH MINDSET: THE KEY TO RESILIENCE

How will you react when you encounter challenges throughout the next year?

The first step in overcoming these emotional challenges is embracing a **growth mindset**. Psychologist Carol Dweck popularized this term in her book *Mindset* and argues that abilities can be developed through hard work, dedication, and learning from mistakes. In contrast, a **fixed mindset** is a belief that intelligence is predetermined and cannot be changed.

Adopting a growth mindset can be transformative for those in medicine. When you encounter a difficult patient case or an unfamiliar procedure, view these as opportunities to grow instead of retreating into self-doubt. Pushing out of your comfort zone won't be easy, but it's a rite of passage we go through.

The takeaway: Listen to your inner dialogue as you encounter challenges and reframe towards the positive. "I can't do this" becomes "I can't do this *yet.*"

REKINDLE YOUR MOTIVATION

The next strategy for overcoming emotional hurdles is "remembering your why." Angela Duckworth highlighted this concept in her bestselling book *Grit.* She recommends tapping into the core reasons that drove you to pursue your career.

Take a moment to reflect on why you chose this path. Was it to help people in their time of need? Was it a personal experience that drew you into healthcare? Whatever your motivation, revisiting these core drivers can help rekindle your passion and provide the strength to overcome this challenging year.

Motivations will be different for everyone, but rest assured, you've chosen a great path. I have loved my medical career, as do countless others. Douglas Wong is a practicing PA who describes his joy in practicing medicine:

"I've worked in a lot of fields. Web Design, IT, Retail, Real Estate, and Education. And the thing I love most about medicine is that almost all my time is spent in the pursuit of making people's lives better.

This happens as a result of my decisions, built upon the edifice of two hundred years of human progress. When I don't have the answer, I can easily turn to the pinnacle of human training in physicians for guidance and teaching.

Human beings and the world we have built are flawed and broken. The decisions we make as a society are wrought with mistakes. But in this role, as a PA, I can be part of the effort to make things a little better. I get to fix things. People get better. That's what I love most."

DOUGLAS WONG, PA-C

The takeaway: Take a moment to revisit your motivations and keep them at the top of your mind when you hit bumps in the road.

BALANCING WORK AND PERSONAL LIFE

Our final strategy is striking a healthy balance between your work and personal life. Medicine envelops people if they aren't careful, quickly leading to burnout.

I learned this the hard way. I enjoyed learning medicine so much that it became a seven-days-a-week endeavor. Before long, the joy of learning medicine faded and my relationship with my family strained to the point that I stopped studying altogether. It took me a while to appreciate the importance of balance.

It's crucial to set boundaries and reserve time for rest. **Designate specific times for self-care activities** that bring you joy, relaxation, and detachment from work. Whether reading a book, practicing yoga, or spending time with loved ones, make these activities a non-negotiable part of your routine.

Moreover, **guard the days off that overlap with your family** and ensure these times are free from work-related discussions. Giving your mind a chance to recharge from the pressures of medicine will significantly boost your resilience and overall mental well-being. Over time, you'll find that this balance leads to increased effectiveness in your work.

The takeaway: Create a schedule that emphasizes relationships and time away from medicine, and stick with it.

LOOKING AHEAD

As you begin this new chapter of your life, you may ask, "When does it get better? When will I start to feel confident?" Here is the short answer: *success breeds confidence.*

You will learn clinical medicine and practice applying it during periods of supervision. After repeatedly seeing successful results, your confidence will naturally set in. Each good outcome will be a brick in your foundation.

The hard part is enduring the early phases until you gain the necessary experience. The question becomes, "Do I have the mental fortitude to endure?"

Pause and take a moment to evaluate your mental well-being. Assess where you stand on the spectrum from healthy stress to maladaptive anxiety. If you find yourself leaning more towards the latter, it's perfectly okay.

· · ·

There are resources available and steps you can take to manage your emotional state better:

- **Embrace your support system:** Start a group text thread with your closest classmates. Reach out to them when you need a boost, share your worries, or enjoy the camaraderie.
- **Tap into your professional network:** Senior colleagues and mentors can provide perspective and guidance. Their reassurances will remind you that what you're going through is a normal part of the journey.
- **Read some perspective-changing books:** Learn from the wisdom of the books mentioned in this chapter — *Mindset* and *Grit*. These resources compile decades of research and offer insights into overcoming emotional challenges.
- **Get professional help if needed:** Cognitive behavioral therapists are experts at helping patients notice when worries become maladaptive and the steps they can take to course-correct. We routinely recommend this to patients, and we can follow our own advice too!

I don't want to suggest that everyone will have universally terrible experiences in their first year. There will be many positive experiences — but you don't need a guidebook for those. My goal here is to equip you with the right mindset so that you'll be ready to handle any challenge that comes your way. As they say, *prepare for the worst and hope for the best*.

CHAPTER 2
GET ORGANIZED FOR SUCCESS WITH GRADUATION CHECKLISTS

BEING well-organized is essential for a smooth transition to practice. Poor organization can lead to missed deadlines, forgotten tasks, and uncompleted paperwork, which can delay your start date and first paycheck. Some of my colleagues have experienced delays of three months or more due to minor oversights that caused them to miss credentialing windows. Using *checklists* can mitigate these risks. I've prepared two checklists to guide you through this next phase.

PRE-GRADUATION CHECKLIST

In the time leading up to your graduation, focus on solidifying your professional network. Complete the following tasks while you still have access to your university email. Once you lose your school email, you will lose access to much of this information. The checklist on the next page is also available for download on my website ClassroomToClinician.com.

NEW PA/NP CHECKLIST
Before graduation

BOARDS EXAM PLANNING

- [ ] **SIGN UP FOR YOUR BOARDS EXAM**. MOST TAKE THEIR EXAMS 2 WEEKS TO 2 MONTHS AFTER GRADUATION.
- [ ] DECIDE ON A **BOARD EXAM STUDY PLAN**.

NETWORK, NETWORK, NETWORK

- [ ] CREATE A **DOCUMENT** WITH THE CONTACT INFORMATION FOR YOUR CLASSMATES, SCHOOL FACULTY, AND PRECEPTORS.
- [ ] UPDATE YOUR **LINKEDIN** PROFILE THEN ADD EVERYONE ABOVE TO YOUR NETWORK.
- [ ] NOTIFY YOUR **PRECEPTORS** ABOUT YOUR JOB SEARCH 4 TO 6 MONTHS BEFORE GRADUATION.
- [ ] FIND 3 WILLING INDIVIDUALS TO BE YOUR **WORK REFERENCES**.

JOB PROSPECTING

- [ ] **EXPLORE** THE JOB MARKET NEAR YOU.
- [ ] START WORKING ON YOUR **JOB APPLICATION MATERIALS**.

FINANCIAL PREPARATION

PREPARE FOR THE **FINANCIAL DROUGHT:** THE 2-6 MONTHS WITHOUT PAY BEFORE YOUR FIRST PAYCHECK. CONSIDER THE FOLLOWING IF YOU PREDICT RUNNING OUT OF FUNDS ---

- [ ] **MAX OUT YOUR STUDENT LOANS** DURING YOUR LAST SEMESTER
- [ ] ASK YOUR FUTURE EMPLOYER (IF ALREADY HIRED) IF THEY CAN OFFER A **LOAN OR ADVANCE** ON YOUR FIRST PAYCHECK.

STEPS AFTER YOU GRADUATE

Once you've graduated, shift your focus to maneuvering through various state and federal licensing procedures. These steps don't need to be completed sequentially, but the state licensing and credentialing steps should be completed as soon as possible.

NEW GRAD CHECKLIST
After graduation (1 of 2)

OBTAIN ESSENTIAL SCHOOL DOCUMENTS

☐ GET COPIES OF YOUR **DIPLOMA** AND SCHOOL **TRANSCRIPTS**

PASS YOUR BOARDS AND NEXT STEPS

☐ EXPECT YOUR EXAM RESULTS IN A FEW WEEKS. AFTER THIS, YOU CAN **REGISTER ON YOUR PROFESSION'S WEBSITE** (E.G., NCCPA.ORG) TO GET YOUR **PROFESSIONAL CERTIFICATE**.

APPLY FOR A NATIONAL PROVIDER IDENTIFIER (NPI) NUMBER

☐ APPLY AT **NPPS.CMS.HHS.GOV.** IMPORTANT: USE YOUR **EMPLOYER'S OR SCHOOL'S ADDRESS**. THIS INFORMATION IS IMMEDIATELY POSTED ONLINE FOR PUBLIC ACCESS, SO DO NOT PUT YOUR PERSONAL PHONE NUMBER OR HOME ADDRESS.

APPLY FOR YOUR STATE MEDICAL/NURSING LICENSE

☐ BEGIN THE ONLINE APPLICATION FOR YOUR **STATE LICENSE** AS SOON AS POSSIBLE, BECAUSE THIS CAN TAKE OVER 3 MONTHS IN SOME STATES. CALL THE LICENSING OFFICE TO SEE IF ANYTHING CAN EXPEDITE THE PROCESS, LIKE SUBMITTING FORMS IN PERSON.

APPLY FOR A DEA LICENSE

☐ APPLY FOR **A DEA LICENSE** *ONLY ONCE YOU HAVE A JOB LINED UP.* THIS REQUIRES A BUSINESS ADDRESS AND TYPICALLY TAKES 1-6 WEEKS TO COMPLETE. SOME STATES WON'T ISSUE IT UNTIL A SUPERVISING PHYSICIAN DELEGATION IS ON RECORD.

☐ SIGN UP FOR YOUR STATE'S **CONTROLLED SUBSTANCE PRESCRIPTION MONITORING PROGRAM** WHERE APPLICABLE. YOUR JOB'S ONBOARDING TEAM CAN HELP DIRECT YOU THROUGH THIS PROCESS.

NEW GRAD CHECKLIST
After graduation (2 of 2)

ENSURE TRAINING AND CERTIFICATIONS ARE UP TO DATE

- [ ] THIS INCLUDES SPECIALTY-SPECIFIC CERTS LIKE **BLS, ACLS, ETC.**

CREDENTIALING AND PRIVILEDGES FOR YOUR FIRST JOB

- [ ] BEGIN THIS PROCESS AS SOON AS POSSIBLE, AS THIS CAN TAKE OVER 4 MONTHS IN SOME HEALTH SYSTEMS. IN ADDITION TO THE DOCUMENTS LISTED ABOVE, THEY OFTEN REQUIRE YOUR **IMMUNIZATION RECORDS** (INCLUDING DEMONSTRATION OF HEP B IMMUNITY).
- [ ] THE ONBOARDING TEAM WILL HELP YOU FILL OUT THE REQUIRED FORMS FOR YOUR STATE, LIKE THE **SUPERVISING/COLLABORATING PHYSICIAN DELEGATION FORMS.**

ADDITIONAL TIPS

- [ ] UPLOAD EVERY IMPORTANT DOCUMENT IN THIS LIST TO **CLOUD STORAGE** TO EASILY SEND THEM TO FUTURE CREDENTIALING TEAMS.
- [ ] **SAVE USERNAMES AND PASSWORDS** FOR THE ABOVE WEBSITES IN A SECURE DOCUMENT.
- [ ] **SAVE RECEIPTS** DURING THIS PROCESS, AS MANY JOBS WILL REIMBURSE THESE EXPENSES RETROACTIVELY.
- [ ] **BE PROACTIVE!** SOME HOSPITAL SYSTEMS ONLY CREDENTIAL DURING LIMITED TIME PERIODS. IF YOU MISS A CREDENTIALING WINDOW, IT CAN DELAY YOURT START DATE BY SEVERAL WEEKS.

With the checklists freeing up some mental bandwidth, you can focus more of your energy on securing your first job. This is an exciting phase, and the next section will prepare you for it.

PART TWO
HOW TO FIND A JOB
WITH GOOD SUPPORT

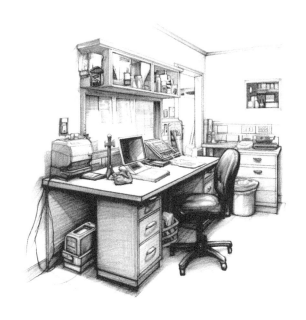

YOUR FIRST JOB

Finding a job with good support is one of the most important things you can do to ensure safe medical practice in your first year. The rest of the book discusses topics like improving your diagnostic and treatment skills. These are great, but they take time to develop. Your employer and attending physician will be your critical safety net from day one while you hone your skills.

Consider this new graduate comparing and contrasting their job with that of a friend:

"My classmate took a job with a hospitalist group that had minimal orientation or training. It was a high-pressure environment, and they managed complex patients independently within a month of starting. They told me about a case of a sick asthmatic who wasn't responding to typical therapy. Their attending was unavailable, as occasionally happened. They felt completely overwhelmed.

In contrast, I found a great job where my group understands the challenges we face as new grads. My attending has an 'open-door policy,' frequently checks in with me, and I get help from experienced nurses too. It feels like I'm part of a team. I recognize that I have a lot to learn, but the pressure isn't all on my shoulders."

Your top priority right now should be finding a job with good support. We will review each step in the job search from start to finish and share concrete advice on achieving this goal.

But prepare yourself — it won't be easy. The job search can feel like an uphill battle for new graduates. Every employer seems to list "two years of experience required." How can you break into your specialty and find a good job?

The next chapters will review the following:

- Choosing a specialty
- The application process
- Creating a compelling CV and Cover Letter
- Acing interviews
- Avoiding red flags

- Seeking positive qualities
- Negotiating a better package
- Deciphering contracts
- Deciding between multiple offers
- Next steps if you don't get any offers

CHAPTER 3
CHOOSE YOUR SPECIALTY

"Hey everyone, I just graduated and took my boards. I've been putting off the decision of picking a specialty, and now I feel lost... I enjoyed most of my rotations and no single specialty jumped out to me as 'the one.' Most job offers around here are for subspecialty jobs, but I've read on forums that people advise against that. What would you all recommend?"

NEW GRAD PA, 2024

YOU CAN'T START your job search until you clarify what specialty you'll pursue. Feel free to skip to the next chapter if you've already decided. If you've been kicking this can down the road, you've now reached the end of the road. It might seem daunting, but a few steps can help you with this decision.

First, take some time to reflect on your rotation experiences:

- **Patient population:** Which types of patients did you enjoy working with the most? Acute or chronic disease management? Do you prefer building long-term relationships or treating patients and moving on?

- **Work environment:** Do you enjoy hospital settings or office-based practices? Do you prefer hands-on procedural medicine or cerebral work?
- **Medical interests:** Which areas of clinical medicine excite you the most? Would you still be excited to grow in the specialty five years from now?

Second, **research your target specialties more**. Our two-month rotations are not long enough to know the realities of every specialty. The following questions — answered via online searches and asking your network — are particularly valuable to the new grad:

- How is the experience for new grads working in this specialty?
- How satisfied are people working in this specialty after five years of practice?
- What is the burnout rate of this specialty?
- Is this specialty generally open to hiring new grads?

Once you've finished your research and reflection, it's time to **assess your findings and decide**. If one specialty stands out as a great fit, follow your gut and go for it!

Many aren't so lucky, and that's okay. For those still unsure, the following advice will help you make this decision —

- **Prefer *broad* specialties over *subspecialized*:** Generalist specialties like family medicine, internal medicine, emergency medicine, trauma surgery, and general surgery will provide long-term career flexibility. If you instead start your career with a hyper-specialized job like sleep medicine, you'll have a much harder time getting out of that specialty later.
- **Narrow to *two or more* specialties instead of *one*:** As long as you're considering broad specialties, applying to jobs across a few specialties will help your search. This leads us to our last point.
- **Prioritize *specific job offers* over the *specialty*:** Your top specialty might be emergency medicine. But if the only offer you can get with excellent training is in critical care — that would serve you much better.

Even if you choose the "wrong specialty," your flexibility as an APP is still much better than that of physicians, so you can always change your mind later. Trust your instincts and don't stress too much about this decision.

———

With your specialty chosen, it's time to ensure that your application materials are up to par. These documents serve as your first impression and are crucial in getting you past the initial screening stage.

CHAPTER 4
OPTIMIZE YOUR APPLICATION

CREATING an outstanding job application is akin to crafting a compelling story — one that tells potential employers where you've been, where you're going, and how you can contribute to their team.

In this chapter, we will dissect the key components of this narrative: your curriculum vitae (CV), cover letter, and professional references. These days, hiring managers may receive dozens of applications for each open role. Let's make your application stand out from the crowd.

ANATOMY OF THE CURRICULUM VITAE (CV)

Your CV is the synopsis of your professional experience. It starts with a succinct **summary statement** (2-3 sentences) articulating who you are and what kind of job you want. Tweak this section to make it specific to the role you're applying for.

Next, detail your **graduate education,** expanding on the experiences *relevant* to the job you are applying for. If you apply to emergency medicine (EM), share your rotation experiences in EM, trauma surgery, and acute care pediatrics. Include any **prior work experience** relevant to the role. These sections are the most essential details to emphasize early in your CV.

The remaining sections should *not* take up prime real estate but should still be included toward the side or bottom:

- **Certifications** you have accrued (e.g., ACLS).
- Relevant **skills** (e.g., bilingual).
- **Professional references** and their contact information.

Last are the *optional* categories to include *if it is relevant* to the job you're applying for:

- **Honors and awards** (e.g., academic achievement scholarships).
- **Research**, **presentations**, **abstracts**, and **publications**.
- **Professional memberships** (e.g., fellow of the Society of Emergency Medicine PAs).
- An **interests section** can include fun facts about yourself to demonstrate your personality and spark conversation during the interview.

————

That is a lot to consider including in your CV! If you're not careful, blindly filling in each section can result in a bloated and bland application that won't get you far. **So, how can you craft a competitive edge over your peers?**

- **Use objective numbers:** Make it clear where you are stronger than the average new grad. If you chose an elective in family medicine and had twice the number of hours as the average student, spell that out. Share the numbers if you performed substantial procedures related to that specialty. However, if the objective numbers don't sound impressive, write that you had the experience and omit the exact number.
- **Highlight relevant work experience:** This is especially true for nurse practitioners who worked as nurses in the same specialty. Employers value this experience, so make it stand out by putting it on the *first page* of your CV.
- **Trim the fat:** The average job applicant has a bloated CV that hasn't been curated to the job they're applying for. Go line by line down your CV and ask yourself if you'd care about it if you were the hiring manager. If not, cut it out.

- **Use keywords from the job posting:** The bigger job boards and HR platforms often use *automated screening programs* to filter applications before they reach human eyes. Including the keywords from the job posting will ensure you make the cut. For instance, the posting might say they're looking for someone who can "complete medical evaluations and EMR documentation" or "work with a diverse patient population." Include a *skills section* of your CV with bullet points for these keywords.
- **Use a sharp-looking professional template:** Those with bland CVs won't get points against their application because that's what we see most commonly from clinicians. However, this is a simple way to stand out because so few people take the time to do this. When I'm reviewing stacks of CVs and I find one that looks great, it sets a great first impression.

On the next page, I'll share my **new grad CV template**. I have posted it on ClassroomToClinician.com under the "Free resources" section. There are many other options for creating professional CVs as well:

- **Canva** has many beautiful CV templates.
- **Freelancers** on platforms like Fiverr[1] can custom-make a CV for under $75.
- **Artificial intelligence (AI) websites** like Rezi.AI, ChatGPT, and KickResume.com can help you write a CV from scratch or revise an existing one.

---

1. "Find Talent To Write Your Resume." Accessed April 4, 2023. https://www.fiverr.com/categories/writing-translation/resume-writing.

JOHN STANGL, PA-C

📞 +917-456-7890

✉️ myemail@gmail.com

📍 123 Anywhere St., NYC

PROFESSIONAL SUMMARY

New graduate physician assistant with years of prior work experience caring for emergency department patients. Seeking an emergency medicine position with a support system for new graduates near my hometown of Seattle.

GRADUATE EDUCATION

University of Wisconsin-Madison

Masters in physician assistant studies: 2013 - 2015
- 2,000+ clinical rotation hours, details below
- Academic honors

Clinical rotation experiences

Emergency medicine
- An elective in addition to core rotation allowed 4 months of EM rotations, averaging 50 hours per week.
  - Evaluated patients and presented to APPs + attending physicians in the main ED.
  - Weekly didactic conference for EM core content, as well as self-study of Tintinelli's Textbook.
  - Proctored procedural experiences:
    - 6 intubations
    - 8 central lines
    - Experience as well with paracentesis, fracture reduction, splinting, suturing, ultrasound and more.

Other relevant rotations
- Trauma surgery
- Pediatric emergency medicine
- Hospitalist medicine
- Medical ICU
- OB-GYN
- Rural family medicine
- Psychiatry

WORK EXPERIENCE

Lead ED Technician

Meriter Hospital, Madison WI: 2009-2013
- 4,000+ hours
- Full breadth of ED tech responsibilities
- Phlebotomy
- Lead training and scheduling

SKILLS

→ Bilingual Spanish
→ Resuscitation
→ Adult + pediatrics
→ Clinical evaluation
→ Lab interpretation
→ Xray interpretation
→ EM procedures
→ Epic EMR

CERTIFICATIONS

NCCPA ID 123456

Active 5/30/2024
Expires 5/30/2034

NPI 123456

Web Design & Development

NY State License

License # 123456
Active 5/1/2024
Expires 5/1/2027

ACLS, BLS, PALS

License # 123456
Active 5/1/2024
Expires 5/1/2027

CV template page 1, available on Classroomtoclinician.com

JOHN STANGL, PA-C

📞 +917-456-7890
✉ myemail@gmail.com
📍 123 Anywhere St., NYC

WORK EXPERIENCE (CONT)

Medical Assistant

Hearth Nursing Homes: 2007-2009
- Dementia unit
- Medication administration

PAST EDUCATION

Central Oregon University

Bachelor of science, clinical physiology: 2009-2013
- Academic honors

WORK REFERENCES

Tody Calogh, PA-C

Tacoma Emergency Care Physicians
305-435-6407. |. tody.calogh@tecp.org

Bill Ding, NP

Tacoma Emergency Care Physicians
305-435-6407. |. tody.calogh@tecp.org

Dr. Pepper

Tacoma Emergency Care Physicians
305-435-6407. |. tody.calogh@tecp.org

INTERESTS

→ Pickleball, semi-professional
→ Bouldering, V4 on a. good day
→ Passionate home cook (award winning chili!)

CV template page 2, available on Classroomtoclinician.com

SECURING STELLAR PROFESSIONAL REFERENCES

If your profile is strong overall, but your reference raises a red flag, it can kill your application on the spot. Reflect on all the people who might be willing references (e.g., preceptors, school faculty, or prior employers), and only choose people who will give you a *raving* review.

You can determine if their review will be positive or negative in two ways. **First, set up a call with them.** Let them know you are looking for jobs and need professional references, and listen to their reaction. Do they immediately volunteer to be your reference, or do they start making excuses about how busy they've been?

If they voice interest, I would ask them, **"Would you be willing to give me a *strong* professional reference? If not, there are no hard feelings, but please let me know now."**

If they pass both tests, you can rest assured they will be a great reference.

————

CRAFTING A CONVINCING COVER LETTER

Your cover letter offers a chance to present your story and highlight your strengths in greater depth. The cover letter should be one page long and include:

- **Your "one-liner":** The first few sentences concisely summarize who you are and what you're looking for.
- **Your reasons for wanting that particular job:** The hiring committee wants to bring on people who will stay long-term. Convince them you have valid reasons to stay. Perhaps the group has an excellent reputation for training new grads, or they're located in your hometown where you have roots that will keep you long-term.
- **"Name-drops":** If you know someone in their group willing to give you a referral, write that you've spoken with them at length about the position and think it would be a great fit. Even if you've just had an introductory call with a practice manager, including their name will demonstrate familiarity with their team.
- **What you can offer their group:** Use this section to highlight your greatest strengths, which might be challenging to do in the CV. You can share these as a few bullet points for ease of reading.

The cover letter I used is shared next. If you like this **template**, you can also find it on my website. AI programs have also helped many with writing and editing their cover letters. Check out AICoverLetter.me and Cover.Doc.ai to generate a cover letter based on the job's unique requirements.

———

Common new grad error: Submitting an application with spelling or grammar errors. Hiring committees sorting through numerous applications will not look kindly on this. **Getting feedback from others is essential.** I recommend the following approach for both your CV and cover letter:

- **First pass:** A basic grammar and spell check with Grammarly premium (free trial available).
- **Second pass:** Get feedback from your closest preceptors and faculty mentors on the application's content.
- **Third pass:** A final grammar and spell check with your loved ones.

If you still aren't happy with your CV or cover letter, here is a new-age suggestion: **Try ChatGPT** with a prompt like the following. I have tried this with impressive results and would encourage you to do the same.

"I would like to improve my cover letter to get an emergency medicine physician assistant job. Please perform a SWOT analysis on my cover letter with specific improvement feedback. After your SWOT analysis, please write an improved version of my cover letter."

Now that your application materials are complete, it's time to apply for jobs!

JOHN STRAFFORD
Physician Assistant

+123-456-7890
callback@gmail.com
123 Anywhere St., New York City

Dr. Helene Paquet
Hiring Manager
Madison Emergency Care Physicians

14th August 2026

Dear Dr. Paquet,

I am truly excited to apply for your physician assistant position with Madison Emergency Care Physicians. I'll graduate from PA school in May and then return to Madison, my hometown. I'm looking to join a team that uses PAs beyond the fast track and fosters a supportive environment for new graduates. After hearing about your group from your lead PA, Jason Morgenstern, it seems like an ideal long-term fit.

I can offer the following strengths to your group:

A well-trained new graduate dedicated to emergency medicine: Einstein Medical Center is home to a busy emergency department and hosts a well-established PA program. By selecting my electives in emergency medicine, I have had extra experiences in the fast track, observation unit, and high-acuity section of the ED. These experiences have fostered a deep-rooted passion for emergency medicine, and I am excited to make this my career.

A bilingual provider fluent in English and Spanish: This skill allows me to provide compassionate, high-quality, and efficient care for our diverse patient population.

A local Madison resident with long-term roots: In discussing with Jason, I know your group has low turnover and values staff retention. MREP sounds like a great practice fit and an ideal location for my family. I grew up down the street from this hospital and would love to make this area my permanent home.

Thank you for this opportunity and for reviewing my application. I look forward to hearing about the next steps.

Sincerely,

John Strafford

CHAPTER 5
NAVIGATE THE JOB SEARCH

THERE ARE countless ways to approach job applications. The key to success lies in your *process* of tackling this challenge. How can you make your process better than the average new grad? Using fishing as an analogy, you can do the following:

- Cast a **medium-sized** net
- Cast it in the **right places**
- Leverage **automated casting technology**

CAST YOUR NET RIGHT

The breadth of your search criteria is essential. Some new grads make the mistake of conducting an excessively broad search, applying to every job they come across regardless of specialty. This approach has many problems, like an application that is too generic to get most jobs.

Others might have an excessively narrow search, applying only to jobs in their dream specialty and dream location. This will limit their chances of finding any offer, much less the perfect one.

The sweet spot is considering jobs in a couple of related specialties in as large a geographic zone as you can tolerate. This is your **medium-sized net**, significantly improving your chances of finding a great position.

————

Next, you'll need to perform that search in the **right places**. If you apply for jobs in the wrong places, you might end up with an exceptionally long job search like what is seen in the Sankey chart below from one new grad:

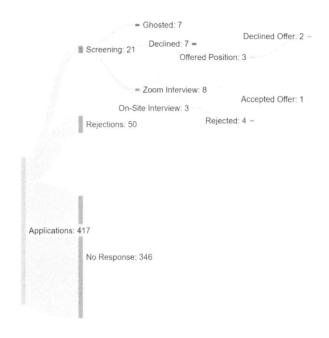

Results from a new grad dermatology job search via a generic job board in 2022, with permission. Generic job boards make it easy to apply to many jobs, but the results are poorer than other means.

So, where are the best places to apply for jobs? I recommend the following step-wise approach:

(1) **Leverage your network.** Start with your network, as they will yield far more than the other options. Contact your preceptors and past employers to ask if their group is hiring. If not, send them your CV and ask them to keep you in mind for future positions. Expand your network by joining local professional organizations for your specialty and attending local conferences.

·   ·   ·

29

(2) **Explore the dedicated websites for local hospitals, clinics, and clinician-owned groups.** Many hospitals and clinics post job openings on their website alone. Since these don't get nearly as many views as the major job boards, your chances will be much higher with these postings. If you are interested in family medicine, try searching for clinics in your area. Bookmark these clinic websites and check their career page regularly. If they don't have any active postings, you can email the practice manager your CV and cover letter to keep on hand should an opening arise.

Most groups only post positions when they have immediate needs, so being among the first few to apply offers a significant advantage. For local groups like this, consider using a **Website Change Detector** like FollowThatPage.com. This will *automatically email you* whenever new posts are added to the "job postings" page, guaranteeing you'll be on the top of the interview pile.

(3) **Job-posting websites.** If you still haven't found a job after the first two steps, broaden your search to the bigger job posting websites. Start with sites specific to the medical community, like the AAPA Job Board, ENP Network, Health eCareers, and PracticeMatch. Facebook even has groups for healthcare job postings. If those don't have relevant job postings, you can search the generic job boards like Indeed, LinkedIn, and Monster. I'd encourage you to apply to positions listed for "Just PAs" and "Just NPs," regardless of your title. These sites make it easy to upload your materials and apply to many jobs simultaneously, but they yield poorer results. Including key terms from their job posting in your resume can help get your application past automated screenings. Set up **alerts to automatically receive new job postings** matching your criteria.

(4) **Recruiters.** I include these lower in the list as they are often tasked with staffing hard-to-fill positions, which are not likely to be a good fit for a new graduate. The exception would be unfilled positions simply because they are rural and might otherwise be a great learning environment. Beware: Once recruiters get your information, they will contact you regularly and for life! Use an email address and Google Voice number specifically for recruiter use.

You have fine-tuned your application, and your dream employer has offered an interview! Let's prepare for the interview next.

CHAPTER 6
ACE THE INTERVIEW

SECURING AN INTERVIEW IS A SIGNIFICANT MILESTONE. It's the final and most important step to land a job offer. While your application was crucial in getting you to this point, the hiring committee makes the decision to hire entirely based on the interview. You'll need to elevate your interviewing skills above your peers to get the best jobs.

Here are the strategies to succeed in the interview phase:

- Learn what **answers** the hiring committees are hoping to hear from new grads.
- **Practice** the list of interview questions ahead of time.
- Before the interview, reflect on **real-life examples** for questions like, "Tell me about a time when you..."
- **Note the most challenging questions**, and consider the STARR framework for these.
- Bring the **printout of questions to ask them** to the interview.
- **Dress for success** and let your **personality show**.

———

WHAT EMPLOYERS WANT

When interviewing new graduates, group managers have specific things they want to confirm:

1. *Do you know what you're getting yourself into?* Interviewers want to hear you understand their specialty's modern-day challenges and are still excited to make this your career. Nobody benefits when a new hire realizes they don't like the specialty and leaves after two months. Articulate your rotation experiences exposed you to these challenges, and you remain passionate about the specialty.
2. *How quickly will you get up and running?* They want to ensure you are "teachable," open to constructive criticism, and actively preparing for the role. Be ready to spell out exactly what steps you're taking to prepare.
3. *Do you know your limits and can ask for help?* Supervising physicians want to ensure you're humble and acknowledge you have much to learn. Emphasize that you'll have no problem asking for help when needed.
4. *Will you be easy to work with, or will you be an "HR problem?"* Groups want that fine balance of professionalism and personality. Dress well for the interview and let your personality show. Demonstrating a positive attitude during the interview will go a long way. Avoid disparaging comments about other professions, like one candidate I interviewed who said, "I became a PA so I wouldn't be overworked and out of shape like doctors." He didn't realize that there was a physician on the interview panel!
5. *How long will you stick around?* They will invest in you as a new graduate and want to be convinced that you have concrete reasons to stay in the area. Share your interest in the group and the region/community.

Our group has something like this in the form of a grading rubric to score candidates in each section. We don't ask these questions directly but use the longer list of questions later in the chapter to make our assessment.

JOB APPLICATION OVERVIEW

01 SUBMIT APPLICATION

02 EMPLOYER RESPONSE
Expect an email or phone call within a few weeks of submitting your job application.

03 PHONE SCREENER
This is often the hiring manager, HR representative, or the company's recruiter to ask screening questions.

04 IN PERSON INTERVIEW
This includes a tour and round-table interview with the practice managers and clinicians.

05 CONTRACT OFFER AND SIGNING
Offers are usually sent within two weeks of the interview.

THE SETTING AND TIMELINE

After submitting your application, the first person to reach out is usually non-clinical, like the office manager, an HR representative, or the company's recruiter. They'll set up a call early in the process to discuss the job's core features and ensure you meet the base qualifications for the role. Afterward, they'll reach out with the next steps for the interview.

The setting for interviews will vary widely. Small community groups might have you speak virtually with one or two people over an app like Zoom before giving you an offer. Other groups might have you come in person with a few other candidates and do rotating interviews with panels of people.

Regardless, the questions will be similar. Preparation is key to performing well in your interview. Try to remember **specific work experiences** that support the points you want to make. Many candidates struggle with questions like, "**Tell me about a time when you** [encountered a challenging patient and how you handled it]." Thinking on the spot about the perfect case is much harder than reflecting ahead of time.

Pretend you are in the moment, dressed professionally, with your physician employer sitting across from you. How will you respond to the following questions? I'd encourage you to answer them out loud by yourself and note the most challenging questions. Take more time to reflect on these, write an outline of how you'd like to answer them, and then practice with friends and family.

––––

Getting to know you

- Tell us your story and what brought you to apply to our job. This is often called your "elevator pitch."
- What do you feel are your strengths and weaknesses?
- How would your coworkers describe your personality?
- Where do you see yourself in five or ten years?
- What are your hobbies or stress relievers?

Your professional experience

- Tell us about your pre-PA/NP school experience.
- How comfortable would you be independently caring for most patients in your specialty?
- Tell us about your procedural experience and comfort level.
- Present an interesting patient case for us, and detail what you learned from that case.

Why this specialty?

- Why did you choose this specialty?
- Tell us about a patient experience that solidified your love of this specialty.
- What have you been doing to study and prepare on your own?
- What are the challenges of this specialty, and how are you planning to overcome them?

Why our group?

- Why did you apply to our group?
- Describe your ideal group or work setting.
- What are your "must haves" or "deal-breakers in a job?"

How would you deal with potential challenges?

- Do you have a plan to manage work-life challenges like burnout?
- Tell us about a time when you failed something and how you responded to that situation.
- What would you do if faced with a moral dilemma (such as your supervisor drinking before working)?
- Tell us about a time when you had a disagreement with a boss at work and how you handled it.
- What would you do if there was a disagreement between you and your attending physician on a clinical situation?
- What would you do if there was personality friction and a nurse regularly delayed performing your orders?
- What will you do if we do not offer a spot in our group?

It is outside this book's scope to give "A+ answers" to every question. Generally speaking, the candidates that stand out the most are the ones who come across as *calm*, *personable*, and *passionate*. Take a deep breath and relax. Don't be afraid to speak casually and say whatever feels natural.

Reflect on what is driving you, and be prepared to share examples that demonstrate your passion for what you do.

Consider using the **STARR framework** for the "behavioral interview questions" that most new grads find challenging. This is a commonly used technique to answer them in a structured way. It stands for situation, task, action, result, and reflection. Here's an example:

Interviewer: "Can you tell me about a time when you faced a challenging patient and how you handled it?"

Situation: "During my clinical rotation in family medicine, I was assigned to a patient who was recently diagnosed with Type 2 diabetes. The patient was upset and struggling to accept the lifestyle changes they would have to make."

Task: "I wanted to provide emotional support, educate the patient, and help them develop a plan to manage their condition."

Action: "I first listened to their concerns and validated their feelings. Then, I used simple language to explain the disease, its complications, and the importance of medications, diet, and exercise. I gave them handouts reviewing what we covered. We set short-term and long-term goals, and I followed up with them regularly to ensure they were making progress."

Result: "Over the next few weeks, the patient gained a better understanding of their condition, became more engaged in managing their diabetes, and showed improvements in their A1C."

Reflection: "This experience taught me the importance of active listening and effective patient education in helping patients cope with challenging diagnoses."

Remember, the interview process is not just about answering questions; it's also your chance to assess whether the group is a good fit and if any **red flags** might be present. The end of the chapter will share a one-pager listing high-yield questions you can bring to the interview. This is also available for download on my website. You don't have to ask every one of these questions, but having them there can spur your memory in an otherwise higher-stress situation.

Below are a few of the questions highlighted in the one-pager. Ask these questions to the interview committee as well as other APPs who work there:

- What are the roles and responsibilities of APPs here?
- How is the workload in patients-per-day, and is it manageable for a new grad?
- How are oversight, education, and mentorship handled?
- How much will support staff help with duties like vitals, rooming, turning over patients, calling patients with test results, etc?
- Can you describe the type of new grad who thrives in this job and the kind who tends to struggle?
- What do clinicians love about working for this company?
- What do they wish they could change?
- What is the average tenure and yearly turnover for the APPs?
- What reasons do people cite when leaving?
- Is there time on-call and what does it entail? What is the pay for it?

Outside of the interview, you will likely be interacting with a representative from the medical group who will explain the other core aspects of the job, such as:

- The pay structure (hourly, salary, overtime pay).
- Whether there is a bonus system or not.
- The schedule, lunch breaks, etc.
- Benefits, like health insurance coverage, 401(k), paid time off (PTO), and paid holidays.
- Continued medical education (CME) allowance.
- Malpractice insurance coverage and whether or not it includes tail coverage.

After the interview concludes, consider sending the interview committee a thank you email in the following days. If you can add a personalized touch specific to each interviewer, that would be even better. Below is a sample of what that might look like.

Dear [Interviewer or Chair of Admissions Committee],

I wanted to thank you and the interview panel for meeting with me. I enjoyed learning more about your position and remain excited about this

opportunity. I was impressed with the [onboarding and training] your group
offers, as it shows how invested you are in APPs.

I look forward to hearing about the next steps. Please do not hesitate to
contact me if I can provide additional information.

Sincerely, [Your name]

These steps collectively ensure you'll be seen as an outstanding candidate and an informed job seeker, improving your chances of landing that dream job.

Key Questions NPs & PAs Should Ask Prospective Employer

Ask these questions during the interview to uncover red flags and positive qualities.

Job-related Questions:

- [ ] What are the clinical responsibilities of the APPs on your staff?
- [ ] Could you provide an idea of the typical workload, including the expected patient rate per hour?
- [ ] What are the non-clinical responsibilities? Any on-call time required?
- [ ] Is there a clearly defined onboarding or training period, and if so, how is it structured?
- [ ] Do you set up new graduates with a senior APP mentor?
- [ ] Can you share an example of something an attending taught an APP in the past week?
- [ ] Can you describe the degree of clinical supervision and oversight?
- [ ] Will I always have access to a senior or supervising physician on-site?
- [ ] What is the ratio of physicians to APPs?
- [ ] What kind of feedback do APPs get on their practice?
- [ ] Are any metrics used to assess our work and productivity, and what are the consequences if these aren't met?
- [ ] What does the work schedule look like, and how is requested time off handled?

Employer and Workplace-Related Questions:

- [ ] Can you share some common positives and negatives that current and past APPs have expressed about working here?
- [ ] What attributes do you believe would increase an applicant's chances of success in this role?
- [ ] Can you tell me why the person who previously held this position left?
- [ ] What are the current staffing needs and the expected start date?
- [ ] Can you share the retention rate or average turnover per year for the APPs and physicians?
- [ ] How well-supported are the APPs and the support staff in your organization?
- [ ] Which Electronic Medical Records (EMR) system do you use?
- [ ] Do you allow double-booking patients in your practice?
- [ ] How has the practice adjusted in response to the COVID-19 pandemic?

Compensation & Benefits Questions (Asked before or after the interview)

- [ ] Could you elaborate on the pay structure, bonus system, and opportunities for overtime?
- [ ] Could you provide an overview of the benefits package, including health insurance, 401(k), PTO, paid holidays, and CME allowance?
- [ ] Can you elaborate on the malpractice insurance coverage, including tail coverage?

Questions for Current and Former APPs Who are NOT on the Interview Committee:

- [ ] What has been your experience working here?
- [ ] What are the clinical roles and responsibilities of the APPs on your staff, and do you feel they are utilized to their full potential?
- [ ] How busy are your days and how easy is it for you to manage your patient load?
- [ ] Can you share some common positives and negatives that the current and past APPs have expressed about working here?
- [ ] Can you tell me why the person who previously held this position left?
- [ ] How was the onboarding and how long was the ramp up period?
- [ ] How well-supported are the APPs, and how well supported is the support staff?
- [ ] Is the practice responsive and supportive if you encounter a difficult or challenging situation?

Questions to Current/Former APPs about the Supervising Physician(s):

- [ ] How often do you have direct contact and communication with your SP?
- [ ] How is it working with your supervising physician?
- [ ] Is the supervising physician kind, patient, and approachable?
- [ ] How busy is their patient panel? Are they easy to ask questions of?
- [ ] Does the supervising physician make a point of teaching? What was the last thing they taught you?
- [ ] How are conflicts or disagreements between the SP and the APP typically handled?

CHAPTER 7
IDENTIFY RED FLAGS AND AVOID TOXIC WORK ENVIRONMENTS

"New grad PA here, almost three months into my first job. Needless to say, this job is not what it was made out to be. It's a specialty I like and can be hard to break into, but the environment and amount of work are overwhelming. There is hardly any time during the day to chart, so I have to do most of it at home. The training has been non-existent - I saw a nearly full schedule entirely on my own five weeks in. My mental health is taking a toll, and I don't know how long I can do this. How can I avoid this next time?"

NEW GRAD, DERMATOLOGY

AT THIS POINT, I've heard so many horror stories of new graduates being promised that "perfect job" during interviews, only to later find themselves overwhelmed in a dangerous position. This chapter will review red flags in detail to help you earlier recognize these types of positions. Consider the following warning signs in each step of your job application process.

Consider it a red flag <u>interview experience</u> if the employer:

- Does not allow you to **speak with the APPs** who currently work there.

- Will only answer some of your questions in writing, and **others can only be answered "over the phone."** Similarly, if they say something like, "My word is my bond," you should run. They are not obligated to follow through on any promise if it isn't in writing.
- Does not tell you the **retention rate** for the staff or the average turnover per year. If you find out that the only APPs they have are new graduates with less than one or two years of experience, that is a big red flag.
- Does not say **why** the person whose role you are filling left.

Consider it a red flag offer if the employer:

- Is unwilling to **list benefits in writing or in the contract.** Similarly, if they do not provide health insurance, consider this a red flag (contractor roles are an exception but should have much higher pay).
- Has **stipulations** that you will only maintain benefits if you maintain a certain billing level.
- Includes a **financial penalty** for leaving before a certain time period, suggesting retention issues.
- Does **not offer any paid time off (PTO)**, citing flexible shift work and grouping shifts to allow short vacations when you want them.
- Does **not offer any allowance for continued medical education (CME)**. Are they truly investing in your growth if not?

Consider it a red flag onboarding period if the employer:

- Has a training period with an **offensively low** training pay rate. One new grad shared they were offered a training rate of seventeen dollars per hour for three months (thank you, next). Similarly, if they say, "You'll be onboarding by acting as a scribe/medical assistant for the supervising physician," this is also a red flag. A few shadow shifts in the very beginning with a lower pay rate is a reasonable ask.

- Does not offer an *explicitly defined* **onboarding or training period**. You need at least a few months of strict supervision and training. If you hear them say, "We need you to hit the ground running," this is a red flag.

Consider it a red flag <u>practice environment</u> if the employer:

- Does not give you **access to a senior clinician or attending physician on-site**. "Doctor always available by phone" is insufficient for the average new graduate.
- Refuses to mention the **expectations for patients per hour** or volume per day. Clarify how long the ramp-up period is before you need to hit the expected patients per hour. It should be a minimum of two months.
- Has **minimal support staff** (e.g., medical assistant, front desk) therefore expecting you to do this work.
- Won't confirm other job details like **on-call time** or **unpaid non-clinical duties**.
- Uses an outdated or uncommon **EMR** - this might decrease your efficiency and result in taking charting home. If it isn't one of the main ones like Epic, ask what EMR they use and Google it to see what people say about it.
- Has a **management or medical director team run by non-clinical staff**. If these people dictate how you provide medical care, they should know how hard your job is and the unique function of APPs.
- Has a head office manager who is the **spouse, sibling, or child** of the supervising physician or the owner. While this might not be universally negative, countless APPs have shared how these setups have resulted in unprofessional nightmares.
- Doesn't have a **formal HR department** or policies for reference. One PA online shared that if they ever had an issue to discuss with HR, they'd have to email a contracted HR agency out of state that never solved any problem.
- Runs what looks like a **specialty "patient mill."** One PA described an example cardiology clinic owned by one physician who was never present. Five APPs staffed the clinic and were expected to churn through patients in fifteen-minute slots for

pre-op clearance. Cardiology patients are older and have complex medical problems, so the setup was a recipe for disaster.

- Allows for **double-booking**, as illustrated by one PA working in family practice below.

"I work at a busy federally qualified health center. I was told there was a low potential for double bookings. I anticipated easing into this challenge with maybe one double book in the morning. Not a chance! After two months, they added three double-booked slots in the AM and three in the PM. The patients here are complex and with many comorbidities. I have to use an interpreter for every other patient. I wish I could quit, but I am stuck in a contract for loan repayment."

In this chapter's stories, both new grads were promised one thing and lived the opposite. You might wonder, *What can I do if hiring managers just tell us what we want to hear? I feel like I can't trust anything they say.*

The most effective way to find out if there are red flags is by **talking with the APPs who currently work there or those who recently left.** Ask the employer to speak with at least two current APPs and **search LinkedIn** for those who worked there in the past.

———

Don't panic if you notice a red flag or two from the list above. Many APPs have great jobs with one of the red flags present. For example, one colleague got a sign-on bonus to work in critical care at a hospital with extensive training and supervision for their first year. There is a reasonable ($5,000) pay-back penalty if they leave before two years. She loves the role and says this "red flag" was understandable, given the group's investment in her.

Although a single red flag doesn't automatically rule out a potential job, a collection of these signals should raise concerns about the work environment.

Having covered potential warning signs, the next chapter will focus on the positive aspects to look out for in a healthy practice environment. These attributes are just as crucial in your search for the perfect fit.

CHAPTER 8
FIND THE IDEAL PRACTICE AND ATTENDING PHYSICIAN

FINDING the right practice environment is fundamental to your professional development as a new clinician. After all, we don't learn medicine in a vacuum but as part of a team. A healthy and supportive environment will exponentially speed up your transition to becoming a skilled clinician.

This chapter will explore what constitutes such environments, their defining qualities, and how to detect these jobs during the interview phase.

THE PERFECT PRACTICE ENVIRONMENT FOR A NEW GRAD INCLUDES:

- **A well-defined and slow ramp-up period**. This should ideally be over six months, where you can start at half the expected rate of a seasoned APP and gradually build up. Slowing down will allow you to look things up as you go, which is essential to providing high-quality care. Ideally, this period would be double-covered, so you present most patients to a senior clinician as you get your feet under you.
- **An established process for training and education.** Most practices don't have time to do one-on-one training with your attending, but if they are invested enough to purchase a virtual "boot camp" course or something similar, that is still a positive

sign. A healthy CME fund ($2,000+ per year) also falls into this category.

- **A system in place to allow clinical practice feedback, adequate supervision, and the ability to ask questions at any time.** Getting feedback on your ideas for patient care is essential to your learning and growth. You can't do this if you are on your own. There should be a senior clinician or collaborating physician on-site at all times early in your career. You will have many questions that are hard to answer on UpToDate, and being able to easily "curbside" your seniors with questions is critical. Some practices have "consultation guidelines" that list high-risk situations that warrant consultation with your attending. These are in place to protect you and should be viewed positively.
- **Emphasis on mentorship and growth.** Having a mentor is essential for new grads. Practices that *facilitate* mentor meetings for you are going to be great places to work.

CHARACTERISTICS OF THE IDEAL COLLABORATING PHYSICIAN:

- **Kind, personable, and respectful.** Reflecting on my favorite attendings over the years, it is always the human factor more than their medical knowledge. They should be someone you see yourself enjoying spending time around.
- **Available.** While this ties in with the personality traits above, it also adds the factor of their practice environment. If your attending is overwhelmed with their own busy panel, even the most well-intentioned physician won't be able to dedicate the time needed to your questions and supervision.
- **Passionate about teaching.** Learning medicine is incredibly challenging when done in isolation. If you can find an attending who knows medicine well, can explain it clearly, and enjoys teaching, your rate of improvement will rise dramatically.

You might wonder how you can know at the interviewing stage if this supervising physician is one of the "good ones?" Here is some advice:

- **Trust your gut.** If something feels right or wrong, it probably is.

- **Ask current and past APPs** about their experience working with them.
- **Listen to their terminology.** If they refer to you as the "midlevel" they need to replace, they probably don't hold APPs in the highest regard.
- **Ask how busy their panel is** and how easy it is for current APPs to staff patients with them.
- **Inquire about their teaching activities** with a question like, "Please share a specific example of teaching you did with one of your staff APPs in the past week."

Let's say you've found the perfect practice environment, and the group gives you an offer. What should you do to make the most of the situation? The following chapter will explore how to navigate job offers effectively.

CHAPTER 9
CHOOSE BETWEEN JOB OFFERS WISELY

ONCE THE INTERVIEW HAS CONCLUDED, anticipate a waiting period of a few weeks as the hiring manager makes a decision. If you receive an offer, take a moment to celebrate this significant achievement! It will feel like a huge weight off your shoulders.

If you are interviewing for multiple jobs, ask if they have *a deadline for accepting offers. Usually, this is a few weeks.* This is a critical time to get as many offers as possible so that you can compare, contrast, and negotiate effectively.

NAVIGATING MULTIPLE OFFERS

Receiving multiple offers is terrific, but you will be left with the "paradox of choice." The most commonly asked questions on online forums are: "Is this a good offer? Which offer should I choose?" I created the scoring rubric at the end of this chapter to simplify this decision and add objectivity to the comparison. It can also give you a sense of where each aspect of your offer fits from strong to weak. The print version of the rubric has a limited resolution; you can find a high-resolution version for download on my website.

WHAT IF I DON'T GET AN OFFER?

My first piece of advice is to *develop a thick skin*. Don't take it personally. Instead, consider it a learning experience. There are a few things that you can do to make the most of the situation.

First, **get feedback from each employer about how you could become a stronger candidate**. You also should take a moment to review your application. Put yourself in the shoes of the interviewers and reflect on whether there are any potential red flags in your application. Ask your friends and family to review your application as well. Make the tweaks to your application while the interview process is still fresh in your mind.

Second, **expand the scope of your job applications.** You might have only been applying to a limited number of jobs based on your target location or specialty. With no offers, you may need to move things from your "must have" to your "nice to have" list. I am referring to the job features like pay, location, specialty, etc. Your chances will rise exponentially if you are willing to move nationwide for a job. After that coveted one to two years of experience, you can always return to your desired location to settle down.

Third, consider **attending a PA/NP residency or fellowship program.** Residencies are programs specifically designed to provide the structure, mentorship, and education required to transition to practice successfully. I am biased in this regard, having attended one and now serving as an assistant program director. I loved the experience and recommend it to many. However, they aren't for everyone. The downside of low pay and low acceptance rates limits many from considering the residency path.

WHEN IS A RESIDENCY RIGHT FOR ME?

For those who can manage the lower pay, deciding whether or not to pursue a residency comes down to three variables:

- What are your goals for your career?
- How deep is your knowledge/skill gap?
- What are the odds you can bridge the gap safely without a residency?

If your goal is to work in low to medium-acuity medicine and you had strong experience before graduate school, you probably won't need a residency program to achieve your goals. If you want to work at the top of your license caring for complex patients and don't have a strong healthcare background, you should absolutely consider a residency program.

If you are considering this option, check out my blog detailing each month in my program.[1] I also wrote a book for those pursuing residency programs: *Ultimate Guide to PA & NP Residency & Fellowship Programs*, available on Amazon.[2] In it, I share everything you need to know about the different program types, how to get accepted, and how to make the most of the experience.

———

While deciding on the best job can be stressful, your time and effort will soon be rewarded. Next, we will review compensation packages and how to negotiate for what you're worth.

1. Physician Assistant Forum. "My EM Residency Experience...," July 24, 2015. https://www.physicianassistantforum.com/topic/18574-my-em-residency-experience/.
2. *The Ultimate Guide To Physician Assistant & Nurse Practitioner Residency & Fellowship Programs: Get Accepted And Succeed In Your Dream Program.* John Stangl, PA-C

New Grad PA & NP Job Offer Grading Rubric:

Rate criteria in the left column (1-4x) based on importance to you. Multiply by the points on the top row. Tally the scores on the right to compare job offers. For instance, if a high salary is a top priority for you and the job pays above $135k, score it as 4x3=12 points.

Criteria You assign 1 – 4x multiplier here	Poor (1 point)	Average (2 points)	Fantastic (3 pts)	Score
Specialty	Pigeon-hole subspecialty you aren't interested in.	Good starting specialty with lateral mobility possible after.	Your target specialty. Difficult to break into.	
Location & Commute	Region you don't want to live. >1hr from work or a stressful commute.	Region you'd enjoy living in. Commute <30 minutes.	Your dream location. Bike to work!	
Total W2 Compensation Package (Including Bonus)	<$50/hr or <$90,000 (AAPA new grad 10th Percentile Data 2023)	$64/hr or $100,000 (AAPA new grad 50th Percentile Data 2023)	$75+/hr or $135,000+ (AAPA new grad 90th Percentile Data 2023)	
CME Fund	$500 or less	$1,000 – 2,000	$3,000+	
Schedule and Shifts	5 days/week and stay late. Regular required nights/weekends.	4-5 days/week. Rare required nights/weekends.	3-4 days/week. No required nights/weekend.	
Paid Time Off (PTO)/Vacation	<2 weeks (10 days)	3-4 weeks (15-20 days)	>5 weeks (25 days)	
Experience of Past APPs and Turnover	Terrible experiences. Nobody stays >1 year.	Good experiences. Multiple APPs have been there for 3+ years.	Raving reviews. Average tenure 3+ years, and multiple over 5 years.	
Clinical Roles and Responsibilities	High stress. 15 min appointments (FM). 3-4 pts per hour (PPH) in EM. No cap on inpatient census, avg 14+ pts (IM).	Manageable stress. 20-30 min appt (FM). 2 PPH (EM). 8-12 inpatient census (IM).	Low stress. 30-40 min appt (FM). 1.5 PPH average (EM). 8 inpatient census cap (IM).	
Non-Clinical Responsibilities & Practice Environment	Required call coverage, unpaid. Cover multiple inboxes. Regular double-booking. No admin/charting time.	Rare required call coverage, paid. Cover your own inbox. Very rare double-booking. Minor admin/charting time.	No required call coverage. No inbox coverage. No double booking. Daily dedicated admin/charting time.	
Group's Reputation and Management Skills	Bad local reputation. Current/prior APPs report: Group doesn't respond to staff's needs.	Good reputation. Group listens and often responds to staff needs.	Great reputation, looks great on the next resume. Group immediately responds to staff's needs	
Orientation, Training, and Ramp-Up Period	"We need you to hit the ground running." No onboarding, ramp-up, or training. Or, if present, has a big "training pay cut"	2-3 months of onboarding and ramp-up. Occasional training. No pay cut during training.	6+ months of onboarding and slow ramp-up of PPH. Double-covered shifts. Dedicated training. No pay cut during this period.	
Collaborating/ Supervising Physician	Off-site and difficult to reach Current/prior APPs report they don't like teaching or explaining things.	On-site and often accessible. Explains rationale and occasional teaching when not too busy.	On-site and always easily accessible. Frequently teaches and offers great explanations to questions.	
Mentorship and Ongoing Education	No mentorship or education provided.	No formal mentorship or education but amenable to helping you as needed.	System in place to pair you with a mentor. Recurring group education in place.	
Pass/Fail Checkboxes:	-Health insurance provided? -Malpractice insurance provided *with tail coverage?*		Total score — >	

CHAPTER 10
BECOME A MASTER NEGOTIATOR

MOST GROUPS WILL HAVE a standardized pay structure for APPs based on experience level, and they will tell you there is no ability to negotiate. They say this hoping candidates will not bring up the topic. Regardless, **you should always try to negotiate.**

Even if they truly can't adjust their core pay structure, they may be able to offer things that wouldn't affect their core salary:

- Sign-on bonus
- Relocation bonus
- Milestone bonus (e.g., one-year-mark bonus)
- Collections (RVU-based) bonus
- Loan repayment or tuition reimbursement
- More CME money or paid CME days off
- More paid time off (PTO) or vacation time
- More administrative time
- Stipend for medical equipment unique to the specialty

It is much easier to request these things if you have some *leverage* supporting your request. You might think you have no bargaining power as a new graduate, but you'd be surprised.

Put yourself in the employer's shoes and reflect on what's persuasive to them. Typically, this includes objective data demonstrating they're below the local rate or something else of value you bring to the table.

For example, if your past work or rotation experience would help you get onboarded faster, this will help their income and bottom line. Similarly, lower staff turnover equates to cost savings for their practice — if you have strong ties to the area and will stay long-term, this is valuable to employers.

Here is a summary of the negotiating power you might have:

- **Multiple job offers**. This is the strongest leverage you can get, so now is the time to apply broadly. You can also share job postings for local groups if the pay is higher.
- **Survey data** showing that local pay rates are higher for new graduates than their offer. You can get the average pay by state and county for free through the U.S. Bureau of Labor Statistics Research Website.[1] Paid options include the American Academy of PAs *Salary Report*[2] and the Medical Group Management Association (MGMA) *DataDive*[3]. These both offer specialty-specific data as well. Doximity, Glassdoor, Salary.com, and PayScale.com are alternatives. One PA even created a crowd-sourced Google Doc for the community[4]!
- **Prior work experience** in the specialty before graduate school, demonstrating you'll have a shorter ramp-up period.
- **Strong ties to the area,** indicating you will stay long-term.
- **Extended vacancy of the position**, which could drive them to improve the package. They are losing money every month the position is left open.

1. "Nurse Practitioners." Accessed April 3, 2023. https://www.bls.gov/oes/current/oes291171.htm#st.

2. AAPA. "2022 AAPA Salary Report." Accessed April 3, 2023. https://www.aapa.org/research/salary-report/.

3. "MGMA | Data | Healthcare Analytics | Benchmarking." Accessed April 3, 2023. https://www.mgma.com/data/landing-pages/mgma-datadive-overview.

4. https://docs.google.com/spreadsheets/d/1bovb3xewzEqhwHmZr63NPimIqHNxk_mcQXEo9nr39mM/edit

Let's bring this together and share how you might negotiate after their initial offer:

You: I appreciate your offer and think the role would be a great fit. However, the compensation is below the typical range for this position. Is there anything you can do to improve it?

Employer: Unfortunately, our pay rates are standardized. This is what all of our new graduates start at.

You: I understand. However, I want to emphasize that I bring several things of value to your group that other new graduates don't. Thanks to my years of prior work experience in this specialty, I'll be able to get up to speed quicker than most. I will also stay long-term, given that I am local to the area with my roots planted here.

Employer: Those are good points. I can't make any promises, but what did you have in mind?

You: I see most positions offering at least $15,000 more than your practice. If you can't add this to the salary because of standardized pay rates, can you consider a sign-on bonus or loan repayment of this amount?

Employer: I will need to take this to the board for approval.

You: No problem, and thank you for considering. I also want to be honest and share that I am in the final stages of interviewing with two local competitors. The've both given me offers that I am also considering. Please let me know what the board says as soon as you hear.

If they call you back with good news for a raised offer that you accept, remember to follow up with a closed-loop communication email to get it all in writing. "I am happy to accept the revised offer we agreed upon over the phone, with the changes including XYZ. Please confirm these details, and I look forward to signing the contract."

As of 2023, no APP position should pay less than $80,000 outside of a true residency experience. With the job demands, debt from training, and the high-risk nature of the profession, most APPs advocate for a minimum salary of $100,000, even for new graduates. This salary is standard for new grads with a normal job working forty hours a week. The pay should be well over the average for those taking on extra responsibilities like weekends, nights, or on-call coverage.

After a conclusion is reached between you and the practice, they will send an updated employment contract. It is important to review this document closely. The next chapter will review the essentials.

CHAPTER 11
DECODE EMPLOYMENT CONTRACTS

EXAMINING employment contracts is daunting for everyone, but it's a crucial step in securing a safe position. You don't want to be one of the recurring posts I see on online forums:

"Help! This job is NOT what I was promised, but now here I am, stuck and unable to get out of the contract without a $10,000 penalty. The hiring team downplayed this possibility, but I wish I had truly understood what I was signing up for."

NEW GRAD, DERMATOLOGY

Understanding employment contracts is a frequently requested topic by new graduates, prompting me to research this topic in-depth and seek the expertise of an industry leader.

Contract Diagnostics is the expert that first came to my mind. I have heard their name repeatedly over the years from my coworkers and in online forums. Their team specializes in physician and APP employment contracts and compensation reviews. Their group includes attorneys, HR professionals, and clinicians. My friends who have worked with them had excellent experiences. The American College of Cardiology has even selected them as their official provider of contract review services.

I reached out to Jon Appino, the company's founder. Jon's mother is a nurse practitioner, so he was excited to support our cause of protecting

APPs from dangerous contracts. I collected the most frequently asked questions and interviewed him, and this chapter will summarize the key things you need to know.

Let's break down the elements of an employment contract and spotlight the red flags in each:

- Non-compete and non-solicitation clauses
- Malpractice insurance
- Contract duration and termination provisions
- Job duties and responsibilities
- Compensation and benefits

NON-COMPETE AND NON-SOLICITATION CLAUSES

The non-compete clause should be carefully structured to protect the employer's **legitimate business interests** (such as patient relationships and confidential business information) **without unfairly restricting the clinician's ability to earn a living.** It should clearly define the **geographic area** and the **duration** the clinician is prohibited from working. Ensure these terms are reasonable and not overly restrictive.

Take this example of a red flag non-compete:

"I recently had a remote job offer from a company with a non-compete clause for 40 miles. Penalties would include 75k in fines for each offense for up to 24 months. The contract stated that the non-compete is in the states where they have clinics and "other states." My lawyer reviewed this and stated they are making it too vague by saying "other states" and not listing the actual locations. We asked them to list the locations, and the practice manager immediately rescinded the offer. Nightmare avoided! I'm making this post as a reminder to look at every word of your contract and contact an attorney if necessary."

The **duration** of non-compete clauses typically ranges from **one to two**

years, with enforcement becoming more difficult for periods exceeding three years.

The **geographic restriction** depends on location. Jon notes, "In Manhattan, a reasonable distance might be fifteen city blocks. In rural regions, the distance could easily extend to fifteen miles or more." Anything beyond a thirty-mile radius is often considered too broad and a red flag. Reflect on how easily you could find another job if this position doesn't work out.

Remember, these are general guidelines. Whether a non-compete clause is enforceable depends on state laws, which vary widely. Some states, like California, generally do not enforce non-compete agreements, while others have specific rules or legal precedents about what's considered reasonable. **As of 2024, the Federal Trade Commission (FTC) shared a new guideline limiting non-competes.** However, several stipulations exclude non-profits and other entities frequently seen in healthcare organizations. Time will tell how this impacts healthcare workers going forward.

If you identify an excessive non-compete, there are a few ways they can be amended:

- **Remove it entirely:** There is no harm in asking them to remove it, especially if you won't have a dedicated patient panel.
- **Narrow the geographic distance and duration**: Adjust their cited numbers to make them more reasonable.
- **Specialty-specific and employer-specific:** This takes vague non-competes and clarifies them to their major competitor in your specialty.
- **Replace it with a "patient advertisement clause:"** This allows you to work for a competitor after leaving, but you can't advertise or solicit your old patients.
- **Dissolution upon contract termination:** Add this provision that renders the non-compete clause void if the employment agreement is terminated without cause by the employer or through circumstances outside the clinician's control.

MALPRACTICE INSURANCE

Always review the **medical malpractice insurance** provided. What are the coverage limits and how does that compare to the average for the specialty? Is it claims-made or occurrence? *Occurrence* is the most expensive for the company, but it will cover you for all malpractice claims even after you leave the practice. The "tail coverage" is inherently included in an occurrence policy.

Claims-made policies, however, will only cover you for a claim while actively working for the company. If you are sued a year after quitting, you are on your own. That's why whenever you see "claims-made," you **must** confirm whether they provide tail coverage via a supplemental policy. Ensure this confirmation is in writing somewhere, ideally in the contract.

Purchasing tail coverage yourself is expensive and a red flag if not included. The rule of thumb is **tail coverage costs around double the annual insurance premium**. The premium depends on your specialty and its risk of litigation. If the yearly premium were $4,000, you'd have to spend $8,000 to purchase your tail coverage.

To summarize, it is best practice to email: *Is the malpractice coverage occurrence or claims made? Is tail covered via the malpractice insurance or not? What are the coverage limits?* Ask to have their answer explicitly stated in your contract.

If you do end up joining this group, ask your practice manager for your "certificate of liability insurance." This is the policy statement your employer gets after they pay the insurance company for your coverage. This document will be in your name and clearly outline whether it's claims made or occurrence, the coverage limits, and the date it is activated/expired. Save this document to cloud storage for future employment, as future credentialing teams often request it.

TERMINATION PROVISIONS

The length of your contract and its renewal terms should be clear. Notice periods and grounds for termination should be explicitly written and reasonable. Here is one relevant example:

"I interviewed for a job the other day and everything sounded great. Then I read their contract and now I'm not so sure. They want 120 days notice for resignation. If you cannot give them the 120 days, you'd owe them $15,000! Their training is minimal, but in the contract they state this money covers what they invest in a new employee. Is this typical?"

The notice period required before leaving their employment can vary significantly based on the employer and the specific role. However, **the typical range is 30-60 days for independent contractors and 60-120 days for employees.** The employer in the example above listed the maximum duration and a huge penalty for leaving early. This is overly restrictive and limits your ability to leave a dangerous position. At the same time, two weeks' notice is too short and also a red flag. If you get fired, you'll want at least a month of income, which the termination duration will guarantee. The sweet spot duration for most APPs would fall somewhere around 60 days.

Next, examine the contract to determine whether it operates on a **"Termination for cause"** or **"Termination without cause"** basis. Termination for cause offers more job security as it requires the employer to demonstrate a valid cause like misconduct.

However, in Jon's experience, most healthcare contracts operate on a termination-without-cause basis. Jon says, "Even if there were a documentable cause to fire you, you and the employer would still prefer a termination without citing a specific cause. That would leave you with a clean record (good for you) and prevents you from suing them (good for them). It's a win-win, and why 98% of the time we see *without cause* setups."

TOPICS OFTEN LEFT OFF EMPLOYMENT CONTRACTS

The contract won't contain every detail of your job, as some things are subject to yearly changes within the company. However, you should still ask to verify the following with other official company documents:

- **Detailed Benefits Information:** While a contract may mention benefits like health insurance, retirement plans, or disability coverage, the specifics are often provided in a separate benefits summary or handbook.
- **Detailed Policies and Procedures:** Many employment practices, such as those related to harassment, leave of absence, grievance

procedures, etc., are standardized across an organization and are documented in a separate employee handbook.

- **Performance Evaluations:** The specifics of how and when performance evaluations will occur are typically not included in the contract.

Here is an example of how you might word an email requesting this information:

"Thank you for sending the contract for my review. I wanted to verify a few more areas before making a decision. Could you send me the company's documents detailing workplace policies, procedures, and other benefits like health insurance? I appreciate your help on this."

RED FLAG IDENTIFIED, NOW WHAT?

If the contract has seemed riddled with red flags, give them that feedback and move on. If the job looks great with only a few smaller issues, you may want to negotiate the contract details.

Having them agree to contract changes verbally or via email is not enough. Appino has experienced situations where the practice manager agreed to a change in the contract over email, but the actual contract wasn't adjusted. The practice later claimed, "The hiring manager did not have that authority; it was not agreed upon in our contract, so we cannot uphold it."

Handwriting changes into a contract also isn't good enough. They can lead to disputes over legibility, interpretation, and whether both parties agreed upon the change.

So, what is the right way to go about it? After identifying a red flag, you'll want to **suggest specific changes** and have those changes **explicitly written into an updated contract.**

This is a great time to involve a contract expert and get their thoughts on the case. Set up a contract review discussion with Jon and his team. After this discussion, Jon suggests you ask the employer for a one-on-one phone call, "I hired an expert who wanted me to clarify a few areas in your contract."

Prepare for the conversation ahead of time. Summarize the solutions that would make the contract acceptable to you. Discuss your concerns clearly and professionally, avoiding accusatory language. Focus instead on seeking a mutually beneficial solution, and be prepared to negotiate on the terms. After coming to a verbal agreement, send a follow-up email summarizing the key changes and saying that you're excited to sign the revised contract as soon as they send it back.

Having an expert like Jon and his team at Contract Diagnostics on your side can be a game-changer. In Jon's words, "Reach out **any time you have a new contract** or are looking to **renegotiate your current contract** after working at a company for more than two years."

If you'd like a free consultation with his team, check out my affiliate link **ContractDiagnostics.com/StanglMedical**. They offer flat rates for your contract review. After using this link, you can request 5% off their usual rate.

CHAPTER 12
ACTION ITEMS

You'll need a great job if you want to practice medicine safely and confidently in your first year. The following action items can help you land that dream job:

- **Create a killer application:** Write a strong CV and cover letter using a professional template, objective numbers, and personalized statements for each job. Convince them you'll want to stay long-term. Get feedback and edits before submission.
- **Cast a medium-sized net:** Apply to jobs in your top few specialties and in as broad of a geographic zone as you can tolerate.
- **Cast the net in the right place**: Apply first within your network, then local group websites, then big national job boards, and last, recruiters.
- **Leverage automated casting technology:** Set up a website change detector and job alerts to be the first to apply to local job postings.
- **Prepare for the interview:** Practice the list of questions with friends and family. Put yourself in the hiring manager's shoes to see if your answers reflect what they're hoping to hear. Think ahead of time about specific life experiences that demonstrate what you want to convey.
- **Seek out red flags:** Use the questions printout during interviews. Don't just ask the biased interview panel — ask other staff APPs or those who recently left.

- **Use the job grading rubric:** This will help you compare job details and identify the strongest offers. When unsure which offer to choose, favor the one with the best support.
- **Negotiate to get the package you deserve:** Use offers from their competitors and other points of value to the employer.
- **Review the contract:** Share it with your colleagues or a contract professional like ContractDiagnostics.com/StanglMedical if there are any concerns. Pay particular attention to the non-compete, malpractice insurance, and termination clause sections.

The only way to extinguish unsafe jobs from the market is to band together as APPs and refuse to accept these offers with red flags. I have a free PDF of these past chapters on my website ClassroomToClinician.com. Feel free to share it with your new grad colleagues so we can spread the word.

With a contract signed by all parties, you can now focus on starting your first job. What does onboarding entail? How can I set good first impressions? The next section will review frequently asked questions so you can prepare effectively.

PART THREE
HOW TO ONBOARD EFFICIENTLY AND DEVELOP RELATIONSHIPS

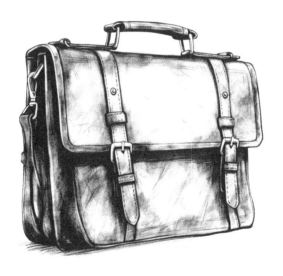

CHAPTER 13
STRATEGIES FOR EFFICIENT ONBOARDING

"I've been so excited to start my first job, but my manager has given me minimal guidance to get up to speed in my first week. I know I'll figure things out eventually, but trial and error on my own has not been fun. My biggest piece of advice to others: find a coworker to be your mentor and iron out the bumps in the beginning."

NEW GRAD NP, 2022

Let's start by congratulating you on your graduation and finding a job. You should feel proud of this accomplishment. Unfortunately, your free time before starting work will pass before you know it, and **onboarding** will be upon you. There are a few key things to do at this stage:

- Learn the specifics about your role and responsibilities.
- Review the policies and procedures of your department.
- Learn the electronic medical records (EMR).
- Set a good first impression with your coworkers.
- Seek out a mentor.

There is a wide range in the quality of onboarding provided by practice managers. Many APPs feel like they are left alone to figure it out. How can you learn this information *efficiently* and acclimate to your new role? This chapter will teach you how to take things into your own hands.

READ WHAT YOU CAN BEFORE STARTING

Before stepping into your new clinic or hospital, try to gain as much insight as possible about your role and responsibilities in this specialty. If your team provides an onboarding packet, read through it before your first day. Two Google searches are also beneficial for new grads:

- "Onboarding guide for PA/NP in [orthopedics]"
- "Intern survival guide in [orthopedics]"

Numerous survival guides for each specialty are posted online for free.[1,2] I first learned about these when I was rotating with physicians who always had a survival guide that they recommended pre-reading before covering a new service. Despite being written by resident physicians, these guides are a great place to start preparing for your first time working in the specialty.

Some managers don't have a set plan for onboarding beyond a day of shadowing and throwing you into the normal workflow. Hopefully you've screened out positions like this during the interview. If not, consider sharing examples online of how other workplaces onboard new APPs. The link below includes a great forum post with dozens of good onboarding examples across multiple specialties.[3]

_____

MAKE A WORK BINDER

You will be given so much information in your first weeks that it will be impossible to memorize. Have a way to collect the many documents and jot down guidance from coworkers. In doing so, you won't have to ask the same questions repeatedly. Another Google search will help you find resources to print before starting:

- "[Rounding notes template/assessment checklists/printout guides] in [internal medicine]"

1. https://www.upstate.edu/medresidency/pdf/UHInternNFSurvivalGuideV4.pdf
2. https://www.hopkinsmedicine.org/-/media/orthopaedic-surgery/documents/resident_survival_guide.pdf
3. https://www.reddit.com/r/medicine/s/HaWf60Zi3a

MedFools.com is one example and shares countless printouts for rounding, assessment, notes, and more. In the next chapter, I'll share one checklist for learning department procedures and EMR actions that you can print before your first day.

————

OVERCOME ONBOARDING CHALLENGES

Even the best jobs will have issues come up during onboarding. **Finding a mentor** is the most helpful way to navigate these challenges. The ideal mentor for you now is not the seasoned APP; **it's the most recent hire to the group**. Ask to schedule a call with them.   All the onboarding roadblocks will be fresh in their minds.

Here are some **high-yield questions** to ask your new co-workers during downtime:

- How was onboarding and ramp-up for you?
- What have you heard are the most frequent challenges/struggles for new hires, and what advice do you have to deal with them?
- What level of independence is expected by each month after orientation?
- What do you wish you knew when you first started?
- When you have clinical questions, what have you found is the best way to get them answered?
- How do our attendings like to hear patient presentations?
- Have you found the group usually liberally orders testing, or are they more stringent?

————

Using these strategies will help you excel on your first days on the job. Next, we will discuss strategies for mastering your department's procedures and using the EMR system effectively.

CHAPTER 14

EMR CRASHCOURSE: STREAMLINE YOUR DAILY PROCESSES

THE ELECTRONIC MEDICAL Records (EMR) system is a mainstay in modern healthcare. It can often seem like an intimidating labyrinth to a new graduate stepping into the world of medicine. Most hospitals will have an EMR training period, but don't expect it to help you much, as the trainers are not specific to your job or department.

This chapter provides a checklist to help you efficiently navigate your EMR and your department's workflows. The document is available on my website for download and printing.

Your coworkers can show you how they accomplish each item from the list:

- Reviewing patient clinical information (test results, prior admissions, etc.).
- Placing orders.
- Writing notes.
- Patient flow through your department.
- Communication with support staff and consultants.
- Gathering supplies for procedures, personal protective equipment, or patient handouts.

Onboarding Checklist For Your First Day

If your employer doesn't have dedicated onboarding aside from having you shadow another provider, try using this checklist on your first days at work for a structured approach. Make sure you know how to accomplish every item from the list and ask your colleagues for help if unsure.

ELECTRONIC MEDICAL RECORDS

Patient Review:
☐ How can you perform "**chart biopsies**," or chart reviews, to find your patient's essential information like past visits, labs, vitals, and imaging reports?

☐ How to use the EMR's **Search function**: What is the most efficient way to find buried information (i.e., past echocardiograms, endoscopies, etc.)?

☐ **Care everywhere**: Where can you find visits and results from other hospitals and providers?

Daily EMR Processes:
☐ **Sign up for a patient**, add them to your rounding list, or find your schedule.

☐ **Put in orders** for diagnostic tests and treatments

☐ **Favorite** individual orders.

☐ Develop your own **order sets**.

☐ Start a new blank note.

☐ How to use a **note template** (and see if they can share a template already used by the group).

☐ **Macros** and dot phrases.

☐ Order **referrals** and give follow-up information to specialists.

☐ Add patient **discharge instructions**.

☐ Input a discharge dot phrase (and see if they can share a templated discharge dot phrase already used by the group)

☐ Get **electronic prescription access** for controlled substances.

ROLES & RESPONSIBILITIES

Department Flow:
☐ Department tour – What is the **patient flow** through their visit? And the **provider workflow**?

Communication:
☐ **How to contact your attending physician:** Would they prefer to be called, texted, or paged?

☐ **What is the preferred way to communicate your needs with support staff:** Verbal, "MD to RN communication" orders in the EMR, or a phone communication system (like Telemediq, Ascom, etc.)?

☐ What are the frequently used phone numbers for the front desk, charge nurse, lab, imaging, and any other department you anticipate needing to contact often?

☐ How to call a specialty **consultation**?

☐ How to contact **ancillary team members** like pharmacy, social work, and other frequently contacted people?

Important Supplies:
☐ **Personal protective equipment (PPE)**, like masks, sterile gloves, etc

☐ **Procedural equipment** – what are the most common procedures done in this setting, and what is needed to get set up for them? Where can I find these items?

☐ **Crash cart** or supplies for patients who decompensate

Provider Resources:
☐ How to access and create an account with **clinical support websites** like UpToDate?

When you are doing your shadowing shifts at the start of your job, there are two important things to help you create a foundation for charting. First, ask for the **note templates** that other APPs use. Second, **keep track of the MRNs of the patients you see while shadowing**. After your shift, you can review their charts to see examples of how your colleagues apply the template to actual patients. Eventually, you can make your own charting style. In your first months, however, it's safest to mimic the style of your coworkers. Since you will access a patient's medical record, remember to ask for their permission while you see them (HIPAA).

———

With the practical onboarding details understood, let's now explore the vital step of establishing a positive relationship with your collaborating physician.

CHAPTER 15

CULTIVATE A GREAT RELATIONSHIP WITH YOUR ATTENDING PHYSICIAN

"My new attending (who I love) described me as being a "1-month-old" in clinician-years. Ha! But as a new grad, I *feel* this in my bones. I'm glad she accepts me as I am and enjoys helping me grow."

NEW GRAD FNP

A HEALTHY RELATIONSHIP with your collaborating or supervising physician (SP) is essential to your successful transition to practice. They will be your primary safety net and teacher during this challenging time.

Many new graduates feel that developing this relationship is more in the hands of their attending, but there is a lot you can do. How can you be the "best new grad" that senior clinicians will enjoy mentoring? One attending physician summarized his thoughts:

"I want new graduates who work hard, ask for help, and try to build rapport with our entire team. I especially love it when they seek to understand *why* we are doing things instead of blindly following orders."

You could even directly ask your attending physician, "Which qualities have you seen in the most successful new APPs in this role?"

Some simple yet powerful attributes can foster a productive relationship with your SP. This chapter will share concrete guidance to help you accomplish this goal.

DEMONSTRATE PROFESSIONALISM

Dress professionally and **arrive five minutes early** to your shifts. Use language appropriate for the workplace and present yourself as a leader for support staff. Avoid using your phone for things like social media while at work.

RESPECT YOUR SENIOR COLLEAGUE'S TIME.

Ask thoughtful questions only after attempting to look up the answer yourself. I found it very helpful to have an app on my phone that stored unanswered questions so that I was always ready to expand my knowledge **when slow moments arose on shift**. Don't ask non-urgent questions during the busiest part of the day.

Keep your patient presentations targeted and concise. Ask your attending up front, "When I present patients to you, do you prefer them to be more concise or thorough?" Alternatively, you can ask, "Generally speaking, do you prefer presentations that last thirty seconds, one minute, or three minutes?"

ACCEPT CRITICISM GRACEFULLY

Take feedback in a **non-confrontational way**. You don't want to challenge your attending or accuse them of being wrong even if you just saw a lecture on the topic by the world's expert. Instead, say, "Yes, I am happy to do that, but can you explain why so I understand the rationale?" The words you use and your body language are essential.

NEVER LIE

Honesty is key. Our residency program always reinforces this critical teaching point: **never lie**. It seems so obvious as not worth mentioning, but you will be surprised at how easily it happens.

Here is an illustrative example: a new grad presented a patient's case who was in an MVC and declared they were "cleared by the Canadian head CT decision rules." When directly asked by the attending, the new grad confirmed they didn't see hemotympanum. However, when the attending examined the patient, the ear canals were occluded with cerumen, so the new grad couldn't have known whether hemotympanum was present.

Put yourself in the shoes of the attending. If you can't trust that 100% of what you are told is accurate, you must repeat the entire H&P on every patient they staff with you. It will be tough to trust them going forward, regardless of whether the misstatement was accidental.

The takeaway: Do not worry about being perceived as not thorough enough if you don't know an answer. You aren't expected to know all the answers. Say, "Great question. I think the answer is X, but I will double-check as soon as we are done talking." Your attendings will be fine with this response. **It is safer to be open about being unsure than over-confident and untrustworthy.**

SHOW YOUR PERSONALITY

Lastly, despite the seriousness of your work, remember to be personable with your colleagues. Strive to create a lighthearted and positive work environment where everyone enjoys working together.

One of my PA friends, Dan, does a great job of this. He keeps a mental note of funny observations at work, which are ubiquitous in medicine. Whenever he walks into the department to start his shift, he greets us and shares a funny story from the past week. This was one of his stories: "I asked my patient if he had any family history of serious conditions, and they said, 'Yes, my mother has cancer, my brother has heart disease, and my dog is on dialysis.'" Every shift working beside Dan is lighthearted and enjoyable.

––––––

Let's next explore how to create a great first impression with the support staff you'll work with daily. Fostering positive relationships with them is as important as your relationship with your attending physician.

CHAPTER 16
SET GOOD FIRST IMPRESSIONS WITH SUPPORT STAFF

IN THE WORLD OF MEDICINE, the saying, "Get on the good side of nursing and support staff—they can make your life heaven or hell," rings particularly true. Sage clinicians emphasize this advice, and my own experience has confirmed its wisdom. I've witnessed abrasive providers ruin relationships with their colleagues through various bad habits such as:

- Not introducing themselves or learning others' names, opting instead for impersonal and commanding expressions like "Nurse!"
- Criticizing staff work with disparaging comments like, "I can't believe they triaged this patient like this—what were they thinking?"
- Dismissively responding to a nurse's concerns or suggestions. As a new grad, if a nurse comes up to you with a thought, you should listen. Even if you disagree, thank them for bringing it to your attention.

Avoid these pitfalls and strive to make a great first impression. The new graduates that the staff loves get welcomed into the work-family with open arms. Remember, they also serve as a safety net for your medical practice.

. . .

Here are some practical strategies to set good first impressions:

- **Introduce yourself:** Go around to meet each staff member in your first days.
- **Remember their names**: This can be challenging if you are covering multiple sites. Ask for the "department's staff photo" and practice everyone's names until it sticks.
- **Set expectations with your coworkers:** "This is my first job as an NP, so I will be slow for a while. I appreciate your patience!"
- **Maintain clear communication:** After you finish your patient evaluation, upon leaving the room, **give the nursing staff a one-liner about what needs to happen.** It could be as simple as saying, "I'm worried about osteomyelitis; they will need a line, labs, and cultures, please." Proactive communication makes the team feel like a unit in sync.
- **Welcome feedback:** Let the nursing staff know you want them to share feedback, concerns, or ideas openly. "Please tell me if you notice me omitting important orders or ordering something that seems wrong."
- **Make life easier for your support staff:** Ask them, "What are the things the clinicians do that grind your gears, and what are the things that I can do to make your life easier?" A classic example is batching the orders you think the patient will need upfront. If you instead "trickle in new orders" every hour because of indecisiveness, their work will increase significantly.

One of the biggest emotional challenges for new graduates is feeling alone and overwhelmed. By following this advice, you'll soon find that you are part of a team there to support you every step of the way. This subtle perspective shift can significantly impact your mental well-being in this challenging phase.

―――――

This concludes the section on onboarding in your first role. Remember, the ultimate goal for this stage is to set up a foundation for success. With the foundation laid, you will now be tasked with a much bigger challenge: patient care and practicing clinical medicine. Do you feel ready to evaluate patients on your own for the first time?

PART FOUR
HOW TO WORKUP PATIENTS EARLY IN YOUR CAREER

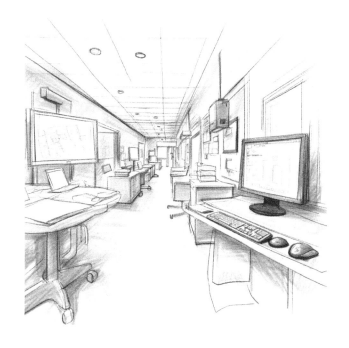

CHAPTER 17
ORDER SETS AND ALGORITHMS

"I remember when first starting, every patient with a chief complaint I hadn't seen before gave ME heartburn. The first time I had a patient complain of hematuria, I had no idea how to work it up.

My life got so much better once I discovered WikEM! I can search Google for "Hematuria WikEM" and get a neatly organized summary with the typical workup. I highly recommend this website to other new grads!"

NEW EM PA-C, 2022

WORKING up patients can feel overwhelming, but we can apply the 80/20 rule. Most workups can be summarized in standard order sets and algorithms for each chief complaint. The challenge is finding reliable and easy-to-use resources. Equipped with these resources, you can quickly start caring for most patients.

Ask your new coworkers what resources they use for order sets and algorithms. This chapter will share general resources that work for most specialties, and the book's last section adds specialty-specific resources.

ORDER SETS BY CHIEF COMPLAINT

Online quick-references:

- Many hospital systems have **built-in order sets in the EMR**. Use those first if they are available.
- **Wikem.org** is an excellent and free reference website run by the UCLA EM residency program. They have countless reference pages for chief complaints and their standard workups.[1]
- **FPNotebook.com** is another free reference that shares typical orders by chief complaint for outpatient providers.[2]
- **PointOfCareMedicine.com** is a free reference for hospital medicine and includes many admission order sets. Check out a screenshot of their workup summaries on the following page.

Print quick-references:

- **EMRA's Basics of EM Pocketbook:** This pocket reference shares the typical DDx and relevant orders to put in for each chief complaint in emergency medicine.
- **Guide to Most Common Internal Medicine Workups**: A highly rated (4.6 stars and over 600 reviews on Amazon) pocket reference for internal medicine.
- **Pocket Primary Care:** A much-loved reference used by many for decades.

As you use these references to place orders, save the orders to your EMR's "favorites" for easy access with future patients.

1. "Acute Chest Pain - WikEM." Accessed March 21, 2023. https://wikem.org/wiki/Acute_chest_pain.
2. "Abdominal Pain Evaluation." Accessed April 11, 2023. https://mobile.fpnotebook.com/Surgery/GI/AbdmnlPnEvltn.htm.

Acute Pancreatitis

Checklist
-- **ABCs:** hypotension/shock, resp distress c/f effusions or ARDS
-- **HPI Intake:** onset, EtOH use, gallstone symptoms, procedures, infectious sxs, family history
-- **Can't Miss:** sepsis, ARDS, hemorrage
-- **Admission Orders:** CXR, strict I/O, decide on bowel rest
-- **Initial Treatment to Consider:** aggressive fluid resuscitation, replete lytes, pain management

Assessment:
-- **History**: *** onset, prior events, EtOH use, gallstone dx, procedures, infectious sxs, FH
-- **Clinical**: *** abd pain, n/v, fevers, constipation
-- **Exam:** *** distress, tachycardia, jaundice, abdominal pain, guarding, flank/umbilical (Grey Turner / Cullen Sign) eccymoses
-- **Data**: *** WBC, lipase, CTAP
-- **Etiology/DDx:** *** EtOH, gallstone, hypertriglyceridemia, anatomic, ERCP, autoimmune, hyperCa

The patient's HPI is notable for ***. Exam showed ***. Labwork and data were notable for ***. Taken together, the patient's presentation is most concerning for ***, with a differential including ***.

Plan:
Workup
-- CBC, BMP (calcium), LFTs (gallstones, cholangitis), coags, lipase, lipid panel (triglyceride) if new diagnosis
-- CXR if dyspneic or c/f ARDS/effusions
-- CTAP with contrast if severe, not sure of diagnosis, or not improving after 48-72hrs
-- RUQUS to rule out gallstones if not EtOH
-- ERCP if gallstone disease; ideally cholecystectomy prior to discharge

Treatment
-- **Fluids:** *** 10mL/kg bolus followed by 1.5cc/kg/hr in first 24 hours
-- **Pain:** *** dilaudid 1mg q4 PRN
-- **Diet:** *** early PO, advance as tolerated; tube feeds if no PO intake at 5-7 days
-- **Nausea**: *** ondansetron 4mg q8 PRN
-- Insulin for hypertriglyceridemia

Sample: Acute pancreatitis summary and order set, PointOfCareMedicine.com

ALGORITHMS TO AID FURTHER WORKUP OF ABNORMAL TEST RESULTS

- **Amboss** is a paid platform with algorithms for common medical workups. @MatthewHoMD is one of the algorithm designers for Amboss and posts his work for free on Twitter. Check out his algorithms for working up low platelets, bleeding, and abnormal PT/PTT.[3,4]

- **Pathway** is another paid program developed to share interactive algorithms to assist patient care.[5]
- **UpToDate** also has many high-quality workup algorithms, though they are typically harder to find within long articles.

COMMON ORDERS FOR EACH SPECIALTY

When I was first starting, I found it helpful to print out a list of the most commonly ordered tests in emergency medicine. Whenever I encountered unclear patient presentations, I could review the list to spark my memory for tests I forgot. I'd encourage you to search online and print a list of your specialty's most commonly ordered tests.

Here is an example list of commonly ordered tests in emergency medicine:

- **Quick bedside testing:** EKG, cardiac monitoring, ETCO2, and fingerstick glucose.
- **Basic labs:** CBC, BMP, LFTs, magnesium, lipase, and HCG.
- **Infectious testing**: UA, lactate, blood cultures, procalcitonin, ESR, CRP, Covid-19 PCR, culture gram stain, and isolation precautions.
- **Cardiovascular:** EKG, troponin, BNP, CXR.
- **Anticoagulation/Hematology:** PT, PTT, type and screen/cross.
- **Imaging:** CXR, CT scan, and bedside US.

IMAGING STUDIES: WHAT TO ORDER WHEN...

For any given chief complaint or diagnosis, you can use online references like the ones found on **Radiax.com or CentralOregonRadiology.com** to see what is likely to be the best starting imaging order to assess that issue.

3. "Evidence-Based Clinical Decision Support." Accessed March 21, 2023. https://www.amboss.com/us/clinicians.

4. Matthew Ho, MD PhD [@MatthewHoMD]. "Consolidated Flowcharts on 1. Approach to Bleeding 2. Working up Thrombocytopenia 3. Working up Elevated PT and/or APTT 4. Working up VWD Https://T.Co/JkRVJb1x9V." Tweet. *Twitter*, February 4, 2023. https://twitter.com/MatthewHoMD/status/1621881585199976452.

5. "Pathway | Rapid & Evidence-Based Decision Support At The Point-Of-Care." Accessed March 21, 2023. https://www.pathway.md/.

UpToDate, WikEM, FPNotebook, and most quick references also offer guidance on this decision.[6,7]

––––––

Order sets, algorithms, and simple references are helpful in the beginning. However, beware that these generic guides are oversimplifications. The patient sitting in front of you will often require more nuanced ordering than what is mentioned.

For example, the Radiax reference says the ideal study for assessing "headache" is CT non-contrast head and MRI brain without contrast. Many patients with headaches do not need advanced imaging. For those with red flags that warrant imaging, our job as clinicians is to assess for the conditions in our differential diagnosis *that might not be found with the typical first-line testing.*

Suppose a patient had a severe headache and was taking estrogen therapy. In that case, our DDx should include things like cerebral venous sinus thrombosis, which could be missed in the studies recommended on the Radiax reference.

Order sets are only meant to address one chief complaint or problem, but patients often have multiple things going on. Creating a problem list will help you add testing and treatment to manage the issues not covered in an order set.

––––––

What other situations require you to deviate from these order sets? The next chapter will review ordering nuance and exceptions in greater depth.

––––––––––––––––

6. Google search "Radiax What to Order When", or hand type: https://www.radiax.com/ portals/1/documents/downloadable%20materials/general%20radia/radiaimctrs_ordering guidef_jun12.pdf
7. Google search "Central Oregon What to Order When", or hand type https:// centraloregonradiology.com/wp-content/uploads/2019/07/REFERRING-PHYSICIAN-REFERENCE-BOOK-Revised-06-01-2019-cdd.pdf

CHAPTER 18

PERSONALIZING ORDER SETS FOR THE PATIENT IN FRONT OF YOU

ORDER SETS ARE useful tools in medical practice. They save time and provide a clear path to start working up a variety of complaints. However, they are not foolproof.

This chapter will discuss two common chief complaints — abdominal pain and chest pain — and their standard order sets. We will explore how adjustments are needed for unique patient scenarios.

You'll note that most changes to the order set are driven by **red flags**, our **differential diagnosis (DDx),** and the patient's **problem list.** Last, we will illustrate the importance of **consulting radiologists** when unsure of the appropriate imaging tests.

Challenge yourself by answering the clinical questions below.

ABDOMINAL PAIN

- What is the standard order set for patients with acute abdominal pain?
- How would you adjust the order set for the following unique scenarios:
- (A) 30-year-old female presenting with acute LLQ abdominal/pelvic region pain and vaginal bleeding + discharge.
- (B) Elderly patient with a history of AFib, presenting with acute onset severe abdominal pain.
- (C) Patient with a history of Roux-en-y gastric bypass presenting with acute abdominal pain.

A standard order set for abdominal pain includes:

- CBC with diff
- BMP or CMP (if LFTs are indicated)
- Lipase (if there's a potential for pancreatitis or biliary pathology)
- HCG (in all childbearing age females)
- Urinalysis
- Imaging (e.g., CT scan or ultrasound) if indicated.

In **scenario (A),** our patient is a female with lower abdominal pain. The standard labs would stay the same, the imaging might start with a pelvic ultrasound, and you might consider a pelvic exam with swabs for STD and vaginitis organisms.

In **scenario (B),** we have an elderly patient with severe abdominal pain. The clinical concern would be vascular pathology like mesenteric ischemia or AAA. Thus you might examine carefully for a AAA, perform a bedside ultrasound, add a lactate, and/or format the imaging as a CT angiogram instead of a typical CT abdomen pelvis with IV contrast.

You might know the contrast is timed to optimize arterial evaluation in a CT angiogram. You wonder if a lack of a venous phased scan limits sensitivity for the rest of the abdominal pathologies. Calling the reading radiologist to discuss questions like this is always worthwhile. Time and time again, they have helped me fine-tune my imaging ordering to ensure I am optimizing my chances of picking up what is going on.

In this case, the technologists can do the angio phasing *and* a venous phase scan, all with the same contrast bolus. Yes, this results in more radiation, but that is less of a concern in these elderly patients with high mortality in acute abdominal pain.

Scenario (C) involves a patient with a history of gastric bypass. Calling the radiologist would help you learn that all bariatric surgery patients should have a short oral contrast prep done just before scanning to assess the surgical site better and improve sensitivity for complications like anastomosis leak, perforation, internal hernia with outlet obstruction, etc.

———

CHEST PAIN

- What is the standard order set for the typical patient with chest pain?
- How would you adjust the orders for the following scenarios?
- (A) A 40-year-old female smoker with chest pain worse with deep breathing, shortness of breath, and sinus tachycardia of 115.
- (B) A 70-year-old male with a history of hypertension presents with chest pain, thoracic back pain with radiation to the L flank, and tingling in his L leg.
- (C) A 45-year-old female with a history of lupus presents with chest pain that is worse with laying flat, with dyspnea on exertion, and you are having difficulty hearing good heart sounds.
- (D) A 60-year-old male with a history of alcohol abuse presents with chest pain and fever after a night of repeated vomiting.

A typical order set for chest pain includes:

- CBC with diff
- BMP or CMP (if LFTs are indicated)
- HCG (in all childbearing-age females)
- EKG
- Troponin
- Chest X-ray

In **scenario (A)** with pleuritic chest pain, we must be suspicious of the possibility of PE. The workup might add a D-dimer or CT angiogram based on their pre-test probability.

In **scenario (B),** recognize that chest pain radiating to the back is a red flag for aortic pathology like aortic dissection, thus necessitating a CT aorta angiogram to the order set.

In **scenario (C),** positional chest pain is concerning for pericarditis and pericardial effusion. Thus, we should scrutinize the EKG and add a bedside ultrasound or formal echocardiogram to assess for pericardial effusion.

In **scenario (D)** with pain after vomiting, consider the possibility of esophageal perforation (Boerhaave's syndrome). If CXR is not definitive, a call with the radiologist could help better clarify the options of CT chest vs esophogram based on your department's capabilities.

————

As you can see, we used red flags, the DDx, and the problem list to adjust our order-set base. If you struggle with these steps, you are not alone. I dedicate an entire book section to leveling up your clinical assessment skills and DDx coming up soon. Before we get to that, the next chapter will share how you can deal with situations of uncertainty when working up patients.

CHAPTER 19
FINDING A BALANCE IN ORDERING TESTS

WHEN YOU HAVE a new patient sitting before you, deciding what tests are needed can be challenging. Admittedly, there is practice variation even amongst experienced clinicians. I've worked with methodical clinicians that incorporate every detail to form a precise DDx and plan. I've also worked with rambunctious ER doctors who refer to their stethoscope as a necklace and have ordered every lab and imaging study before even seeing their patients.

Where should you sit in the spectrum? I'd argue that you should **err towards over-testing** early in your career. After gaining experience, you can **reel it back** to the truly indicated tests.

OVER-TEST TO PROTECT

Why should you over-test early in your career? For one, you are inexperienced, and **your history and physical exam are not fully developed yet**. Adding testing may improve your detection of pathology.

Also, **patients often don't present as the textbook suggests**. Just because a patient has pain in the right upper quadrant (RUQ) doesn't mean they can't have appendicitis. Have a low threshold to work up patients for *higher risk* conditions even if they do not match the classic patient presentation.

Last, **if you *or* your patient are worried about a condition, just order the test**. Your stress level as a new graduate is high enough. Don't lose sleep over this decision.

THE DOWN-SIDES OF EXCESSIVE TESTING

After gaining clinical experience, you will find that reeling in unnecessary testing will make your life easier without sacrificing the quality of care. Why would that make life easier?

Increased testing leads to "**incidentalomas**" you must deal with. This would include incidental lung nodules, isolated elevated bilirubin, and countless more. Unexpected findings are not a benign phenomenon. They often lead to advanced imaging (with its associated radiation), invasive biopsies, and increased stress for patients who now fear things that might never have any consequence.

Over-ordering testing can sometimes paradoxically increase your risk of litigation. I once worked with a very "risk-averse" clinician who liberally ordered non-contrast CT scans on most patients who came to the emergency department (ED) with headaches. If the CT came back negative, he would discharge them.

If he were to have a headache patient with a bad outcome, his practice pattern would likely make him more liable. The standard practice is *not* to routinely image headache patients without red flags. So, his ordering a CT scan tells other clinicians that this patient had a concerning headache. However, a non-contrast CT scan is not sensitive to rule out most conditions on the DDx for emergent headaches, especially if done after six hours from the onset. When you go down this pathway, you often need to follow it with more testing, like a CT angiogram, a lumbar puncture, etc. If you are concerned about a patient, it's better to ask for help from your attending than over-order testing that lacks sensitivity.

During surge season, when the healthcare system is overwhelmed with an influx in patient volume, there will be **pressure to avoid unnecessary testing**. There might be a shortage of testing reagents or prolonged turn-around time for routine testing. You need a solid understanding of the guidelines and indications for testing.

Last, you will soon discover how much of a microscope we can be under as APPs. Physicians on social media and physician organizations **point out that APPs are more likely to order unnecessary testing than physicians**, increasing costs to patients and healthcare systems. Our reputation is on the line, and we must do our part to avoid unnecessary testing.

THE TAKEAWAY

Despite the valid reasons to avoid over-testing, I still recommend erring towards over-testing during the earliest part of your career for the reasons mentioned. Everyone, your colleagues included, will expect you to liberally order tests at first. When you find yourself waffling back and forth on whether something is indicated, just order it!

TRANSITIONING TO JUDICIOUS TESTING

With time, you will learn the techniques to order less without sacrificing quality care. Let's preview a few of these techniques.

First, **ask what the patient's goals are**. I have had countless patients present with severe pain all over the body after a car accident, to the point where if I were to work them up, it would require a head-to-toe scan. However, when I asked them what their goal was for coming, they admitted, "Oh, I just wanted to have this documented for insurance purposes. I feel better now and would prefer to avoid testing if needed." A million-dollar workup was successfully avoided with one simple question.

Second, **pause before ordering each test and ask yourself what you will do with the results**. If it comes back positive or negative, will it change your plan? **If it won't change management, you can probably defer it.** Classic examples include things that are "clinically diagnosed," like displaced nasal bone fractures. Immediate imaging is rarely needed as the diagnosis and initial treatment can be determined by exam alone.

Third, use **shared decision-making** or **informed decision-making**. This is particularly useful in grey-zone situations with no right or wrong answer. Inform the patient of this grey zone, the risks of the pathologies on the DDx that can't be ruled out on clinical exam alone, and the tests available to further delineate things.

Some patients are risk averse and want all the testing immediately. Many others are comfortable living with some risk and prefer the *test of time* instead. If (1) you have a low pre-test suspicion for serious pathology, (2) they can safely follow return precautions, and (3) you document well, you will likely be protected even when deferring testing.

Last, **clinical decision rules** are very helpful in ruling out many conditions without testing. Consider a patient who presents after a head injury and you are considering whether they need a head CT scan. Use an app like *MD-Calc* to review the "Canadian CT head rule," which states that patients who meet several criteria can be safely ruled out from any serious injury without the need for a CT scan. Documenting your review of the decision rule is defensible, and patients will be happy they can avoid a trip to the ED.

Other commonly used decision rules include the PECARN head injury criteria for children, the Canadian C-spine rule, and the PERC criteria for ruling out pulmonary embolism. Decision rules should not be used until you've studied and thoroughly understand each, as novice clinicians might not realize the limitations/pitfalls of each decision rule. You'll need to verify the decision rule has been externally validated and that the patient in front of you matches the inclusion criteria without any exclusion criteria. The PERC rule, for example, should only be applied to *low-risk* patients, as determined by something like the Well's score for objective risk stratification.

———

This chapter concludes the introduction to working up patients. We have applied the 80/20 rule and focused on the bare minimum knowledge and resources to get you to a beginner level of function. Now it's time to take your clinical evaluation skills to the next level.

PART FIVE

HOW TO LEVEL UP YOUR CLINICAL EVALUATION SKILLS

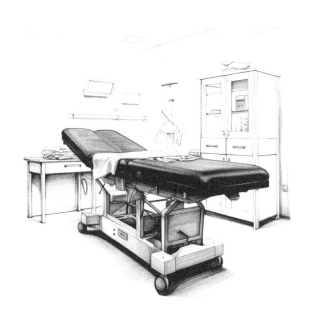

CLINICAL PROBLEM SOLVING

"Our NP program has been lacking in connecting our didactic content with diagnostic reasoning. Our professors ask us to memorize lists of diagnoses, symptoms, and treatments on a PowerPoint deck.

New NPs need frameworks to help us incorporate our clinical findings and test results into the bigger picture. We need to see how we use the information to develop a differential diagnosis and reach the final diagnosis. Our program let us down in this regard."

SENIOR NP STUDENT, 2023

This graduating student demonstrates impressive insight in the excerpt above. While many students focus on passing a test, she wants to apply this knowledge to her future patients.

While some patients present to you as if they "walked right out of the textbook," the majority are not so straightforward. Most modern patients have extensive past medical histories and multiple complaints.

Imagine sitting in front of a 57-year-old woman who checked in with complaints of anxiety, shortness of breath, headache, tingling in her feet, high blood pressure readings at home, and oddly colored stools. How would you sort all of this out?

You are tasked with remembering the appropriate questions to ask, exam maneuvers to do, differential diagnoses to consider, tests to order, and much more. In the moment, it can feel like an amorphous swirl of countless things to cover.

Luckily, there are several things you can do to improve your patient assessment skills. The following chapters will break down each step of clinical evaluation so you can evaluate patients confidently and improve your diagnosis rate.

We will review the following strategies, all of which can be implemented on your next clinical shift:

- Determine whether your patient is an **"ABC or H&P patient."**
- Use a **systematic approach** for each patient, with a **checklist-style printout** if needed.

- Use a **prompt system** to remember what assessments to perform.
- **Improve your DDx** creation using techniques like SPIT.
- Pause to **review data,** sort into **signal vs noise**, and make a **problem list.**
- Make a **summary statement** focusing on the strongest signals to guide the next steps.
- Consider **admission versus discharge criteria** for every patient.

The Patient Assessment

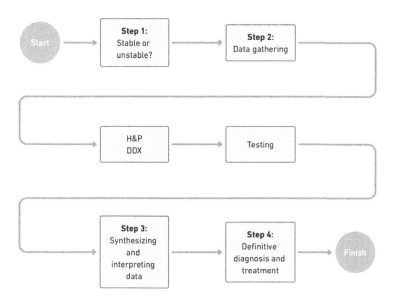

CHAPTER 20
STEP 1: DETERMINE STABILITY

DETERMINING stability is the crucial first step in your clinical evaluation because it forms the first key branch point: **"Is this an H&P patient or an ABC patient?"** In other words, is this someone who you have time to do the systematic evaluation for, or do you need to focus immediately on resuscitation?

For patients who are unstable, the approach is **flipped**: they require *empiric treatment* and disposition *before* a thorough history, physical, and testing. This concept is well explained in the YouTube video "Emergency Thinking" by Dr. Reuben Strayer. It is mandatory viewing for our APP residents.

So, how do you determine if a patient is unstable or acutely sick?

I like the approach put forth by the APPs that host the "Critical Care Scenarios" podcast:

---

(1) Stable or unstable is primarily a function of the patient's **vital signs**: Hypotension, hypoxia, tachycardia (~120+), or tachypnea (~25+) are all indicators for an unstable patient. Beware the respiratory rate recorded on the chart, as this is notorious for being guesstimated by support staff doing a three-second inspection.

(2) Sick or not sick is a function of the rapid bedside **exam** of the **ABCDs**. It is often apparent as you walk into the exam room:

From the doorway, how does their **airway** and **breathing** look? Are they sitting bolt upright, tripoding, and showing retractions? If so, they are probably sick and need immediate therapy.

To assess **circulation**, observe the patient and put your hands on their extremities. Are they pale, cold, clammy/diaphoretic, or mottled? All are concerning features.

For **disability** assessment, observe them during your initial interactions. Do they have a depressed mental status? Are they awake and interacting appropriately?

Sick patients might have normal vital signs but can be picked up with this brief ABCD exam.

If you get the sense that your patient is unstable or sick, there are a few things you need to do immediately:

- **Find your nursing staff and communicate** that this patient needs help.
- **Start resuscitation** (e.g., fluids, medications).
- **Notify your attending physician**.
- **Seek transfer to a higher level of care.**

———

If your patient is stable, as is the case for most of our encounters, you can continue down the usual steps in the clinical encounter. We will review these in the next chapters.

CHAPTER 21
STEP 2A: BACKGROUND REVIEW

"I started my first job about a month ago. Every time I walk in to see a patient, my mind seems to blank. I forget some of the important questions to ask and exam maneuvers to do. I use references to remind me, but I still forget some things even if I review them right before entering the room. I wonder, how do experienced APPs keep it all straight?"

NEW GRAD PA, FM

IN THE SECOND step of the clinical encounter, we seek out all the data needed to make a definitive diagnosis. This "data-gathering" refers to many things:

- Interviewing the patient.
- Performing a physical exam.
- Ordering diagnostic tests.

As noted in the excerpt above, this step is challenging for new grads. How do experienced clinicians do it?

We utilize the **same process** for every patient to ensure we never miss important details. We systematically review the patient's **background** information and **foreground** complaints. We use **prompts** to guide groups of questions that logically make sense. In doing so, we don't need to rote memorize a list of seemingly random questions. We make mental notes of any **problems** as we hear them, which guides our testing and **summary statement.**

Let's explore these bolded topics further...

STEP 2(A): THE INITIAL HISTORY AND PHYSICAL

I want to first emphasize the importance of reviewing every patient's **background** health information. Our morbidity and mortality committee has seen numerous poor outcomes after a new clinician focused only on the patient's presenting complaints.

Here is an illustrative case: A new graduate APP was working in the fast track of the ED when they saw a 60-year-old patient complaining of "popping a pimple" on their leg with resultant cellulitis. He had normal vital signs, and he looked well overall. It seemed like an open-shut case, and the APP prescribed cephalexin and TMP-Sulfa to the patient. The patient bounced back several days later with an intracranial hemorrhage and an INR through the roof. The patient was new to their system and had no background information on their chart. The APP didn't habitually ask every patient about background conditions and medications. Otherwise, they would have discovered his history of atrial fibrillation for which he takes warfarin, highly interacting with TMP-Sulfa.

The background review doesn't have to be a long process in which you review every medical detail dating back decades. However, you should review the patient's chart on the computer and ask the patient about *active high-risk* medical problems:

Past medical history (PMH): *"Do you have any serious medical problems? Or, what medical problems do you take medication for?"*

Be sure to make special note of any high-risk conditions, like **vascular** disease, **organ failure** (e.g., cirrhosis, ESRD, CHF), **immunocompromised** state, **hyper-coagulable state**, or another condition prone to **complications** (e.g., cancer, neutropenia, pulmonary hypertension, endocrinopathy like adrenal insufficiency, and myasthenia gravis).

Past surgical history (PSH): *"Have you had any big surgeries before?"*

Make a note of the surgeries that put them at risk of complications for the rest of their life, like cardiovascular surgery (CABG, aortic repair, valvular repair), bariatric surgery, transplant patients, splenectomy, or device/hardware (LVAD, VP shunt).

Medications: *"What medications are you taking now?"*

Hopefully, they don't respond with the classic, "I'm taking two yellow pills, a big square one, and a blue one, but I'm sure you can sort it out from that." If they do, ask to have their family send a picture. Note the medications that put them at risk for complications, like anticoagulation (warfarin, DOACs), chemotherapy and biologics, chronic steroids, and oral contraceptive medications.

Social history (SH): *"Any drug or alcohol use?"*

Note the high-risk social activities, like alcoholism, IV drug abuse, homelessness, etc.

Graduating students frequently tell me, "I still don't understand what is considered *relevant* background information to include in presentations." The answer to their question is the list above.

As a new grad, make note whenever your patients have one of these higher-risk background conditions. These guide testing and should be included in your case presentations.

With the patient's background conditions well understood, we can now focus on evaluating the patient's new complaints.

CHAPTER 22
STEP 2B: FOREGROUND ASSESSMENT

WE'VE NOW REACHED the point where the patient tells us their story and reason for seeking care. This is the pivotal point where most diagnoses are made. We call this the foreground, which refers to everything surrounding the patient's current illness:

- The chief complaint (CC) and history of present illness (HPI)
- The review of systems (ROS)
- The physical exam
- The diagnostic test results

———

The history and physical section is broken down into two basic steps.

First, in a **"patient-centered"** part of the interview, we let them tell us their story in their own words using open-ended questions. Two areas from their story need to be clarified up front: the *tempo* of the illness and *what has been done thus far* by prior clinicians.

As the master diagnostician Dr. Rabih Geha says, **"Tempo is queen"** and should be clarified because it helps us immediately narrow the potential causes. Ask your patients, "When and how did your symptoms first start, and how quickly have they progressed?"

A sudden or hyper-acute onset of symptoms occurs over a period of seconds to minutes. It is high risk as it only occurs with a limited number of concerning possibilities:

- **Vascular pathologies:** blockages (e.g., arterial occlusion), bleeds (e.g., subarachnoid hemorrhage), dissections, or ruptures (e.g., aortic aneurysm rupture).
- **Electrical activity** (e.g., seizure, dysrhythmia).
- **Blockages** (e.g., kidney stone or gallstone pancreatitis) or **perforations** (perforated bowel).
- **Rapid action of a specific drug or medication** (e.g., an overdose of insulin or opiates.

Acute onset refers to symptoms developing over hours to days and adds infectious, inflammatory, and toxic-metabolic possibilities. Subacute and chronic tempo add rheumatological, endocrine, and neoplastic conditions. You can listen to Rabih (@rabihmgeha on Twitter) apply this concept to real patient cases on his *Clinical Problem Solvers* platform via the Podcast App. I'll share more on this fantastic resource in a few chapters.

———

In the second part of the patient interview, we have the **"clinician-centered"** section, where we perform targeted history and exam maneuvers to answer *our* questions. We must know how to approach each chief complaint and assess for red flags. Internalizing these things takes time, study, and experience. Let's review a system many experienced clinicians use to remember everything during the evaluation.

THE "BATCHED" H&P

Suppose you are assessing a middle-aged patient with hemoptysis. How many pertinent questions and exam maneuvers can you come up with? Many new grads struggle to memorize "the thirty things to assess in patients with hemoptysis" listed in traditional textbook chapters.

Most experienced clinicians haven't memorized such a list. They ask batches of questions based on *prompts* that they give themselves. They remember their assessment for hemoptysis using the prompts **Background-Foreground-DDx-Testing-Treatment-Disposition** as follows:

Background-related prompts: You consider if there is anything in this patient's background history that might be related — "Have you ever had hemoptysis before? Are you taking blood thinners?"

Foreground-related questions: You can use clarifying questions like those from the OLDCARTs or PQRST framework frequently taught in school.[1] As you study the approach to each chief complaint, your targeted questions and red flag evaluation fall into this prompt. An example of one of these questions would be, "What are the associated signs and symptoms you've had with the hemoptysis? Have you had pain anywhere? Are you short of breath?"

DDx-related prompts: You go line by line down your working DDx, using each condition to remember more batches of questions.

Pulmonary embolism — You pull up MD Calc on your phone and review Wells and PERC criteria, asking, "Have you ever had a DVT, PE, or increased clotting condition? Do you take estrogens? Any recent surgery or immobilization? Are the associated signs and symptoms consistent with PE? Is the chest pain pleuritic? Is there associated dyspnea?" Also, assess the vital signs and examine for findings consistent with PE, like tachycardia, JVD, leg swelling, etc. Don't feel bad about using a phone to reference things like MD Calc, even while in the room with the patient.

Tuberculosis — "Have you ever lived outside the US (if so, where?) or been exposed to people with known TB? Have you had a chronic cough? Have you had any night sweats, weight loss, etc.?"

Lung cancer — "Have you had a smoking history?"

Testing-based prompts: You consider the various tests that might be ordered for this complaint and ask questions to help narrow down the best test. In this case, you might consider a CXR or a chest CT scan. Your review of the Wells and PERC criteria can be applied to sort out the best test.

Treatment-based prompts: You consider the various treatments that might be helpful for this problem. For example, what situations with

---

1. REAL First Aid. "The Art of Questioning - PQRST." Accessed March 3, 2023. https:// www.realfirstaid.co.uk/pqrst.

hemoptysis might benefit from antibiotics? This would prompt a batch of questions assessing if the hemoptysis might be from pneumonia or a COPD exacerbation — "Have you had any fevers, productive cough, history of smoking, COPD, or wheezing?"

Disposition-based prompts: You look into the future and consider whether the patient will be safe to go home or need admission. What information will you need to make that call? In this case, it would prompt me to examine her ambulatory pulse oximetry. If she is hypoxic, we know she will likely need admission unless she significantly improves after our treatment.

You won't necessarily have to use every prompt for straightforward cases. However, they are beneficial with complex patients and those in whom you feel you're forgetting things.

PHYSICAL EXAM PEARLS

Three teaching points are essential for new clinicians to develop an effective physical exam. First, always **undress your patients** and inspect the skin in the area of their concern. You'll undoubtedly find patients with a "strained back" that has a skin rash consistent with shingles.

If they are having pain, **have them point** specifically to the point of maximal pain. Many patients who are checked into our system with a complaint of back pain actually have flank pain, with a completely different DDx and approach. Similarly, patients might report lower chest pain when, on the exam, they point at and have tenderness to the abdomen's RUQ.

Last, use a **"hypothesis-driven"** physical exam instead of a general head-to-toe screening exam. The problem with a generic screening exam is that "the eye doesn't see what the mind isn't looking for." Your rate of detecting a subtle murmur will be much higher when faced with a febrile IV drug user that you're worried might have endocarditis and specifically seek out the murmur. The more specific your questions and concerns, the better your exam will be. A famous article from the rational clinical exam series further illustrates this point: "Does my patient with liver disease have cirrhosis?"[2] By assessing for exam findings that suggest portal hypertension (e.g., caput medusa) and hyperestrogenism (e.g., palmar erythema and gynecomastia), you can make significant progress in answering this question.

———

Notice that the **DDx** helped us the most to focus our assessment in both the prompt system and the physical exam. How can you make a strong DDx for any given patient? Let's review this next.

2. Udell JA, Wang CS, Tinmouth J, et al. Does This Patient With Liver Disease Have Cirrhosis? JAMA. 2012;307(8):832–842. doi:10.1001/jama.2012.186

CHAPTER 23
STEP 2C: TOOLKITS TO CRAFT A DDX

"As a new graduate, I've struggled with making a solid differential diagnosis. I often gather the history, do an exam, and come up with the likely diagnosis, but I have difficulty seeing anything other than that. I recognize that I have an issue with anchoring bias and would love tips to overcome it."

NEW GRAD PA, IM

CREATING strong differential diagnoses (DDx) is essential to practice medicine safely. A weak DDx can result in dangerous cognitive errors like **anchoring bias** and **premature closure bias.** With both of these biases, the clinician prematurely "anchors" on their first impression, to the point that they put excessive weight on the data that support their belief and ignore data that suggest a different cause.

An illustrative case went through my morbidity and mortality (M&M) committee: a 61-year-old woman with a history of smoking, COPD, HTN, and HLD presented to her primary care APP complaining of shortness of breath and coughing that worsened when she laid flat. The APP suspected pneumonia and prescribed an antibiotic. The patient returned twice after failing to improve and was given different antibiotics both times. The patient eventually went to the ED, where they diagnosed her with decompensated heart failure from a missed myocardial infarction.

A pause for reflection where you consider, "What else might this be?"

is critically important and protects you from these pitfalls. The mere act of creating a DDx ensures you take that pause.

While everyone recognizes the importance of the DDx, it still isn't easy to create them. Many new grads feel this is a major weakness and something they want to improve upon. I recommend a targeted approach. Two considerations will guide your DDx for any given patient: the **risk** of the situation and the **number of complaints.**

This chapter will share strategies to deal with each variation —

- Low-risk situation: **SPIT** out a quick DDx
- High-risk situation: Add in **VINDICATE** or external resources like **diagnostic schemas.**
- Multiple complaints: Try the **ChatGPT** DDx generator.

———

LOW-RISK SITUATIONS: USE THE SPIT TECHNIQUE

You don't need to generate an expansive DDx when dealing with most healthy patients with straightforward symptoms. Instead, a concise DDx is most effective. Use the "SPIT" mnemonic as your guide:

- <u>S</u> - **Serious** — the conditions with the highest morbidity/mortality.
- <u>P</u> - **Probable** — the conditions you think are most likely based on the presentation.
- <u>I</u>- **Interesting** — those esoteric diseases we learned about in school… Could these symptoms align with any of those conditions?
- <u>T</u> - **Treatable** — could this be a condition that would benefit from treatment, like antibiotics?

The clinician considers the clinical picture, and off the top of their head, they quickly generate at least one condition for each SPIT letter. When evaluating an infant with cough, congestion, and wheezing, the SPIT method might generate:

- Serious = congenital heart disease, heart failure, airway obstruction from epiglottitis, or swallowed foreign body.
- Probable = bronchiolitis.
- Interesting = airway malformation/stenosis
- Treatable = pneumonia.

You then consider whether the serious conditions are consistent with the patient's presentation. If not, you can move on. Having at least considered them is the important thing.

HIGH-RISK SITUATIONS: ADD IN VINDICATE AND/OR EXTERNAL RESOURCES

When dealing with high-risk patients or situations, like elderly patients with coexisting conditions or patients who bounced back after treatment failure, you'll want to expand your DDx beyond what immediately jumped out at you. There are a few effective ways to accomplish that.

(1) You can brainstorm yourself using the "**VINDICATE**" mnemonic as a memory aid:

- **V** - Vascular
- **I** - Infectious or Inflammatory
- **N** - Neoplastic (cancer)
- **D** - Deficiency (diet/vitamin), Degeneration, Drugs
- **I** - Intoxication, Iatrogenic, or Idiopathic
- **C** - Congenital
- **A** - Allergy, Autoimmune, Anatomical
- **T** - Traumatic
- **E** - Endocrine and Environmental

The clinician writes as many conditions as possible with each body system as a prompt.

(2) You can also use an "external brain" to help you. The following are some examples of DDx generators for a given chief complaint:

- **Diagnosaurus** differential generator (App and website)

- **UpToDate.com**
- **Wikem.org**
- **Google search** (we've all done it… because it works.)

These external references are great at generating a broad differential diagnosis list. However, you should be mindful of the pitfalls of a DDx that gets too long.

An expansive DDx list suggests the same relative weight for each diagnosis. Epidemiology is not listed, so a new clinician might equally consider a "zebra" when the "horse" five lines down is much more likely. Similarly, the "never-miss" diagnoses can be overlooked in long lists.

Moreover, these long lists don't guide how you should approach the patient. Considering a list of one hundred diagnoses that could cause dyspnea won't inform your next steps.

(3) Many clinical reasoning experts recommend **"diagnostic schemas"** to address these issues. The best schemas attempt to simplify the possible causes into overarching groups of conditions, highlighting which conditions are the most likely and most dangerous. The lists are also organized in a way that guides testing. I advise new grads to reference online schemas whenever they aren't sure of what is happening with a patient and want an actionable DDx reference.

I have found that the *Clinical Problem Solvers* internal medicine education group shares the best free schemas for countless chief complaints and clinical problems.[1] Below are two examples of their schemas for the chief complaint of dyspnea. On their podcast, attendings work through patient cases out loud using these schemas to simplify the approach to challenging patients.

---

1. https://clinicalproblemsolving.com/reasoning-content/

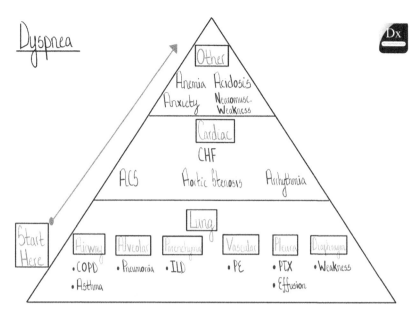

Start your assessment of dyspnea for lung causes, as they are the most common. If no cause is apparent, next inquire about cardiac causes of dyspnea, followed by the rarer causes last.

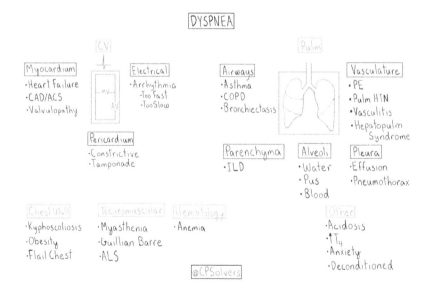

CP Solvers Dyspnea Pyramid, Drs Geha and Manesh, with permission.

MULTIPLE COMPLAINTS: TRY CHATGPT FOR A DDX GENERATOR

Another challenging scenario in creating a DDx arises when a patient presents with multiple complaints. Picture this: a patient has three chief complaints, seven positive Review of Systems (ROS), and five abnormal findings during the physical exam. Using the reference materials we discussed above for each complaint will lead to an impractically time-consuming process.

You should still SPIT out a quick DDx with your initial thoughts. After that, consider giving ChatGPT a try. This AI-based tool from OpenAI can generate a unique DDx based on multiple inputs, acting as your co-pilot and helping you brainstorm more ideas for your targeted DDx.

I have the ChatGPT app on my phone and have experimented with impressive results. Check out this example:

Prompt: "Share a DDx for a patient presenting with chest pain, shortness of breath, hemoptysis, cough, and right leg swelling. Break down the list into common causes and dangerous causes."

ChatGPT:

"Common causes:

(1) Pneumonia: A lung infection that can cause chest pain, shortness of breath, cough, and sometimes hemoptysis.

(2) Acute bronchitis: Inflammation of the bronchial tubes, causing chest pain, shortness of breath, cough, and sometimes hemoptysis.

Dangerous causes:

(1) Pulmonary embolism (PE): A life-threatening condition in which a blood clot from a DVT or another part of the body blocks one or more lung arteries. Symptoms include chest pain, shortness of breath, cough, hemoptysis, and leg swelling.

(2) Congestive heart failure (CHF): A condition in which the heart cannot pump blood effectively, leading to fluid buildup in the lungs and other parts of the body. Symptoms may include chest pain, shortness of breath, cough, and leg swelling.

(3) Lung cancer: A malignant tumor in the lung, which may cause chest pain, persistent cough, hemoptysis, shortness of breath, and sometimes leg swelling due to lymphatic or vascular obstruction.

[…]

AI hasn't made it to the point of replacing your judgment or your attending physician's input in challenging cases. Its use for generating a DDx and clinical decision-making is still experimental and cannot be relied upon. It is prone to blatant errors ("hallucinations") in which it will confidently and persuasively share incorrect information. I consider it helpful in brainstorming but not as a definitive answer. However, it has proven incredibly handy so far on shift and has even passed all of the USMLE exams required of physicians![2] AI will undoubtedly change the face of healthcare in the next decade.

———

With our working DDx formed, we will next place orders for diagnostic testing to arrive at a definitive diagnosis.

2. Kung, Tiffany H., Morgan Cheatham, Arielle Medenilla, Czarina Sillos, Lorie De Leon, Camille Elepaño, Maria Madriaga, et al. "Performance of ChatGPT on USMLE: Potential for AI-Assisted Medical Education Using Large Language Models." *PLOS Digital Health* 2, no. 2 (February 9, 2023): e0000198. https://doi.org/10.1371/journal.pdig.0000198.

CHAPTER 24

STEP 2D: PUTTING IN ORDERS

THE BOOK'S prior section discussed basic order sets you can use based on the patient's chief complaint, but what about everything else your patient has going on? The **problem list** will be your guide. Including a problem list in your approach will ensure you don't miss out on any orders not covered by your order sets.

Let's take a moment to review the stage we are at and how our problem list is formed:

- We've started the data-gathering process with a targeted history and physical exam.
- We've made a working DDx.
- While working through the first two steps, we have jotted down the most important **data points, red flags, and problems** as we hear them. These form our problem list.

Below is an example of what this preliminary problem list (bolded) might look like for a hypothetical case of a middle-aged woman presenting with pleuritic chest pain. We again organize our thinking with the prompt system. Notice how the problem list guides our orders.

Foreground: **Chest pain** —> I will order the standard chest pain order set (i.e., CBC, BMP, EKG, troponin, and CXR).

Background: History of **smoking** and **oral contraceptive use** —> I will add D-dimer and CTA PE protocol if positive. She also has a PMHx of **autoimmune disease** —> I will scrutinize the EKG for pericarditis and consider a bedside ultrasound for a pericardial effusion. The patient is a **female** of reproductive age —> I will check an HCG and hold on imaging until the test results.

DDx/Testing: I reflect on other things on the DDx that might be missed with standard cardiac testing, like an aortic dissection and Boerhave's —> I did not appreciate red flags for these on H&P, but I will scrutinize the CXR.

Treatment: **Symptom control** —> I will offer Tylenol and escalate if needed.

Disposition and other problems identified: She is **homeless** and without health insurance —> will place a consult order for the social worker for follow-up resources if testing is negative.

Once you've ordered everything that comes to mind, **pause for another moment of disposition thinking** related to test results. Ask yourself, "If these tests come back negative, will I feel comfortable with this patient being discharged? Or would I feel uneasy and want even more testing before feeling reassured?"

This prompt requires understanding the **sensitivity** of the tests we order. Ordering a low-sensitivity test with a weak negative predictive value will not help you rule out conditions on your DDx. It's worth considering definitive testing right from the beginning.

I recently saw a patient who illustrated this point. The patient, an active IV drug user, presented with non-traumatic back pain, radiating pain with numbness down his right leg, and tachycardia. Initially, I considered ordering a CBC and CMP, planning to reassess his symptoms after pain management. However, realizing that a normal CBC and CMP wouldn't assure me enough to discharge him, I ordered the spine MRI upfront, which confirmed a spinal epidural abscess (SEA).

With the above approach, you will have ordered the correct tests and will soon have their results. How do we make sense of everything and work towards a final diagnosis? The next chapter will review medical decision-making.

CHAPTER 25
STEP 3A: MEDICAL DECISION MAKING

Evaluating patients can be an absolute nightmare at times. We have to untangle a convoluted history with 90% nonsensical information that does not pertain to the problem at hand. I feel like we need to be a medical detective honing in on the clues for the case, but it sure isn't easy!

EM PA-C

THE THIRD STEP of the patient encounter encompasses the critical thinking needed to reach a diagnosis. It is another common source of stress and errors for new graduates. We are tasked with:

- (A) reviewing *all* of the data.
- (B) determining which *subset* of that data will help us reach a final diagnosis.
- (C) formulating a concise *summary statement* that guides the final evaluation steps.

An essential skill in this step is sorting the **"signal from the noise."**

What do I mean by this? We call abnormal data points "signals" when they help us make progress toward a definitive diagnosis. Examples of signal data points would include RLQ pain with a positive obturator sign and a positive CT scan for appendicitis. The positive CT scan is the strongest signal because it has the highest positive predictive value.

We refer to "noise" data points as those unlikely to be related to the current illness (incidental findings) or those that do not help guide the clinician further (nonspecific findings). Examples of "noise" data points include a complaint of chronic fatigue or test results like a solitary pulmonary nodule.

Challenge yourself with this practice case. Circle what you think are the signals and put an "X" over the noise.

Chief complaint: abdominal pain.

"I've been dealing with some stomach cramps that come and go, and sometimes it hurts to stand up straight. Occasionally I feel bloated and gassy after meals, which can be really uncomfortable. Maybe it's what I eat? I eat a lot of meat and potatoes and not much veggies. I've noticed some dry itchy skin, which I'm not sure is related or not, but I've had that my whole life. I've also had headaches for years now and nobody can figure those out either.

My bowel habits have been all over the place recently too; one day will be normal, and the next day I have several episodes of watery diarrhea. I've noticed some red blood in my stool several times now, which really freaked me out. I'm proud of myself, though, because I have finally managed to lose some weight. I haven't changed my diet or exercised, so I'm not sure how I managed it.

Sometimes I also get these painful cramps in my lower abdomen, and they don't seem to be linked to the bloating. I've also been feeling tired, like I'm always running on empty. A few days ago, I even had a fever of 100.3 and chills."

It's okay if you aren't sure what to make of each complaint. There are some rules of thumb that can help guide you. In general, a symptom or finding is more likely to be a **signal** if it is:

- The patient's **chief complaint.**
- A complaint **in a patient with high-risk comorbidities.** Take every symptom seriously in your vasculopathic patients!

- An **objective finding** (e.g., an abnormal vital sign like fever, or an objective deficit like Babinski sign, etc.).
- A finding with **high specificity or positive predictive value (PPV)** (e.g., elevated lipase for pancreatitis or a "pathognomonic exam finding" like an S3 gallop for CHF).
- A **unique or bizarre finding**, like "purple urine," is probably a signal with a narrow focus.
- A symptom that came on **hyper-acutely** (abrupt onset) given that these tend to come from sinister causes.
- A sign or symptom that is **progressively worsening** over time.
- A **red flag sign or symptom.**
- A part of **an illness' typical presentation**. This ties in with developing pattern recognition skills.
- A **direct temporal association** between their symptoms and a triggering event, and thus reason to consider causation. For example, a patient who reports developing vomiting, paresthesias, bradycardia, and hot/cold temperature reversal that started while eating seafood would be a strong signal for ciguatera poisoning.

For new grads wondering what HPI details to include in presentations: it's anything that fits these criteria!

I want to point out one notable exception to the last bullet point. Patients will frequently share what *they think* is the trigger for their symptoms, but these can often mislead you. If the elderly man says he "strained his back from mowing the lawn," but the back pain didn't start until several hours *after* he finished mowing the lawn, you should categorize the reported "lawn injury" as noise and try to find a serious cause for his back pain. If he said that he felt his bicep pop and swell while lifting the lawnmower into his truck, this direct temporal association would strongly signal a musculoskeletal injury.

On the other hand, an abnormal finding might be **noise** and not helpful in determining the diagnosis if:

- The symptom or sign is entirely **subjective** (e.g., the young and healthy patient with a pan-positive review of systems but nothing objectively abnormal on the exam).

- The symptom is incredibly **nonspecific** (e.g., fatigue or generalized weakness, which does not have much diagnostic specificity).
- It is a **chronic** complaint or finding and is **unchanged** during the current presentation.
- You **can't think of any way** this data point could relate to the clinical picture. For example, consider the patient with a fever and cough who notes "fingernail issues" on the ROS. Since you can't think of any way that could be related to their main issue, it might just be noise.

Just because we have identified an abnormality as "noise," it doesn't mean it can be entirely ignored. Incidental findings like a solitary lung nodule on CXR must be relayed to the patient and given a follow-up plan. However, they shouldn't be included in a summary statement in your presentation.

––––––

Let's apply these concepts. Here is a commonly reported challenge for new graduates:

"Every day, I see a few patients who seem to have a pan-positive review of systems. Neurological complaints like numbness, tingling, and generalized weakness are the most frustrating. It could be nothing at all or something terrible. How do you approach these situations?"

Here is my advice — **seek out the signals:**

- Do they have any high-risk PMH or risk factors?
- Did the symptoms come on suddenly, or are they progressively worsening?
- Are any red flags present (e.g., bowel or bladder involvement)?
- Are there any objective findings on exam?
- Does the clinical picture fit any disease's typical presentation?

I recently saw a patient that brought this to life. She was a middle-aged woman complaining of back pain, fatigue, generalized weakness, stiffness, and tingling in her left leg. She suffered from these symptoms on and off for years. At one point she had a negative lumbar MRI, and since then, was always brushed off to the point where she thought it was all in her head.

I sought objective findings and found them — she was hyper-reflexic on her deep tendon reflexes in her arms and legs. She also had a positive Babinski and Hoffman sign. These upper motor neuron findings suggested a problem above her lumbar spine, and her MRI demonstrated spinal cord changes consistent with multiple sclerosis.

She later sent me a note saying how much her life had improved since starting appropriate medication. A simple neurological exam looking for objective deficits can make all the difference for these patients.

The takeaway: In patients with multiple complaints that paint a complicated picture, try to seek out the signals listed above.

———

TOO MANY SIGNALS!

What about the other end of the spectrum? Whereas some patients have abundant noise, others have numerous abnormalities that fit the signal characteristics above. Consider the elderly patient with numerous high-risk background medical problems, acute-onset complaints, and every test result is abnormal. How can you make progress toward the final diagnosis?

You'll now have to sort the strength of the signals. Start with the **most severe or striking abnormality** to serve as the center of gravity for solving the case. Consider the patient with several abnormal labs, but the most deranged is a calcium level of 16. I write this down and circle it on a piece of paper.

Below it, I write a checklist of another set of findings with the question, **"Of all the signals I've identified, which ones absolutely require an explanation by the end of the case?"** Circle these as well. There will often be soft signals that are not particularly helpful. Sinus tachycardia is one example — it's an objective finding we can't ignore, but it's non-specific. I'll note it mentally but prioritize writing down the patient's petechial rash that always requires an explanation. This reflective question allows me to sort and prioritize the most critical signals.

Now that we have sifted through all the data and identified which are crucial to solving the case, let's learn how to summarize them into a problem statement.

CHAPTER 26
STEP 3B: FRAME THE PROBLEM STATEMENT

"A problem well-stated is a problem half-solved."

*CHARLES KETTERING, INVENTOR AND HEAD OF
RESEARCH FOR GENERAL MOTORS*

I LOVE THIS QUOTE, and it is so well applied to this step of the clinical encounter. Some call this step the summary statement, problem statement, problem representation, or the clinical framing of a case. They all reflect one idea: How can we distill the case's key features into one concise statement that informs the next steps? It generally includes a few things:

- The patient's *age*, *chief complaint*, and *tempo* of illness.
- The *strongest signals* you have identified from the data thus far.
- The *clinical problem* you are left with and how you plan to solve it.

The importance of creating a good summary statement cannot be overstated. The best practitioners are masterful at concisely summarizing complex situations. Merely practicing this skill will help you grow as a clinician. So far, we have covered the first two bullet points. Now, let's focus on how to refine the patient's clinical problem.

When I listen to Rabih and Reza's podcast, I frequently hear them say, "I've heard the patient's story and exam, but I still feel like we haven't clarified the problem we are trying to solve." They are referring to the process of converting *unrefined data* into clinically meaningful problems.

A classic example is the patient who complains of vertigo. Dizziness can be immensely broad, but after our data-gathering phase, we should now refine that complaint into one of the three main buckets of vertigo presentations. Each of these categories has a limited DDx and clear next steps that are supported by leaders in the research of vertigo:[1]

- Triggered episodic vestibular syndrome (e.g., BPPV)
- Spontaneous episodic vestibular syndrome (e.g., Meniere's)
- Acute persistent vestibular syndrome (e.g., Vestibular neuritis or cerebellar stroke)

A patient I saw recently also illustrated this theme. She presented with a chief complaint of dyspnea, which is too vague of a problem to solve. Her CXR, however, demonstrated a cavitary lung lesion. The problem I was then solving was the *cavitary lung lesion* with its much more narrow DDx (e.g., infection like lung abscess, infarct after PE, aspiration, cancer, etc.) and protocol-driven next steps.[2]

Sometimes, our testing comes back largely negative, but that also helps us refine the clinical problem we are trying to solve. Let's go back to our case example of the middle-aged female with chest pain to illustrate what the summary statement might look like:

"This middle-aged homeless woman presents with acute onset chest pain, stable vital signs, and a negative cardiac workup with EKG troponin and CXR. However, she has multiple risk factors for DVT/PE and a positive D-dimer. Thus, our leading concern is a PE. We will proceed with a CTA PE study to further evaluate this possibility."

The problem statement is *constantly re-framed* as we continue through the case. If the above patient's CTA came back negative, the problem

1. Newman-Toker DE, Edlow JA. TiTrATE: A Novel, Evidence-Based Approach to Diagnosing Acute Dizziness and Vertigo. Neurol Clin. 2015 Aug;33(3):577-99, viii. doi: 10.1016/j.ncl.2015.04.011. PMID: 26231273; PMCID: PMC4522574.
2. https://www.the-hospitalist.org/hospitalist/article/35676/pulmonology/best-approach-to-a-cavitary-lung-lesion-update/

statement would again be reframed into a more concise discharge statement with the definitive test results up front:

"We have a middle-aged woman with chest pain and negative cardiac testing plus a negative CTA, with no evidence of an alternative emergency. We will have her follow up in the cardiology clinic to consider stress testing."

This patient case example is just one of countless patient presentations. The challenge lies in the fact that every patient is unique, and framing the problem statement effectively for each patient is very difficult. Improving these skills will take time and experience. However, you can cut down on this time by taking matters into your own hands. The following actions will help you level up your clinical problem-solving skills...

1. LEARN FROM THE MASTERS

Drs. Rabih Geha and Reza Manesh founded the Clinical Problem Solvers and run a premium "RLR podcast.[3]" They dissect challenging core content, teach clinical reasoning, and practice applying it to real patient cases while sharing their thoughts out loud. These two are absolute experts and are by far the best teachers of this material. I learn more in thirty minutes with them than with any other teaching resource! They are double-boarded in EM and IM, have experience working both in clinics and in hospitals, and invite multiple subspecialists to their program. They provide great learning content for most specialties.

Dr. Gurpreet Dhaliwal is another leader in the field. He is an internal medicine professor at UCSF and gives actionable advice in his grand rounds talk, "Clinical Reasoning: Good to Great."[4] He trained Rabih and Reza and they consider him their mentor.

2. REVIEW CHALLENGING CASES WITH A MENTOR

Save challenging patients to a dedicated list in your EMR. Write down

---

3. RLRcpsolvers.com
4. *Clinical Reasoning: Good to Great*, 2016. https://www.youtube.com/watch?v=Qhayc-bRH5g.

what step in the process caused the most confusion. Identify any gaps in knowledge or in problem-solving skills. Then, during your mentor sessions, ask for feedback and compare your mentor's approach with your own. Getting feedback on your critical thinking is essential to fine-tune your skills. Clinicians who have regular self-audits with case logs grow substantially more than those who don't.

3. PRACTICE CLINICAL REASONING WITH SIMULATED CASES

There are many great options for challenging yourself with practice cases. Pretending you're in the moment caring for these patients will help you identify weaknesses and get immediate feedback.

All of the following resources will help your clinical reasoning grow substantially:

- **Podcasts with interactive cases:** EM Clerkship case episodes, EM:Crit's shadowboxing episodes, CoreIM's clinical unknown episodes, and the CP Solvers all do an excellent job presenting challenging patient cases in an interactive way. My favorite cases come from the RLR CP solvers podcast. Pause the episode after they share each aliquot of information. Verbalize your thoughts, summary statement, and the next steps you'd take. Compare your plan with the experts'. Once you get the hang of it, consider joining the CP Solvers live (and free) education sessions where listeners are encouraged to participate.
- **Medical simulation apps:** Apps like HumanDx, Full Code Medical Simulation, FullCodePro, and many others offer fantastic interactive patient cases. They force you to think critically and decide next steps in management. At the end, they grade your decisions, offer case feedback, and share teaching points.
- **Clinical reasoning textbooks:** Dr. Paul Cutler wrote the classic textbook *Problem Solving in Clinical Medicine* in the 1970s, and it remains a treasure. I highly recommend it to anyone who enjoys reading expert physicians work through real patient cases and apply deductive reasoning, much like Sherlock Holmes. A brilliant internal medicine textbook is *Frameworks for Internal*

Medicine by Dr. Mansoor. This book breaks down core content in a way that helps us frame patient presentations logically.

I recognize that there isn't enough time in the year to do everything listed above. Pick and choose whatever fits your learning style best and integrate it into your study routine. Most stressful situations originate from challenging decision-making, so developing these skills will pay dividends in the long term.

––––––

The last consideration of medical decision-making involves disposition planning, which we will review next.

CHAPTER 27
DISPOSITION: ADMIT OR DISCHARGE?

THE PATIENT'S disposition is the ultimate decision point for us. Even if we aren't sure of the final diagnosis or the treatment plan, we must know if it's safe for the patient to go home or not. This is a unique step of medical decision-making that requires its own dedicated pause for reflection.

For the subset of patients with a definitive diagnosis, it's best to find admission criteria for that condition somewhere online like WikEM.org. However, others might have negative testing, but you still don't feel right sending them home. An elderly patient with an ankle sprain and negative X-rays who can't walk would be one example.

This chapter will review general guidelines to help you determine the patient's disposition after your visit. In addition to your usual care, you should assess their updated vital signs, whether they can eat or drink, and what kind of social situation they will face if discharged (living situation, support, and ability to get to appointments). Each case must be considered individually. Don't forget to involve your supervising physician if you are unsure.

In general, you should have a lower threshold to admit if:

- **Admission criteria are met** (on a reference like UpToDate or Wikem.org).
- The illness is **higher severity by risk calculators** (e.g., Curb-65 or PORT score for pneumonia).
- The patient requires **medications that can only be given by IV.**

- The patient is **unable to ambulate** unassisted and is a fall risk.
- The patient has persistently **abnormal vital signs.** (i.e., hypotension, persistent unexplained tachycardia, hypoxia with ambulation trial, etc.).
- The patient requires **close monitoring** (e.g., tongue swelling in angioedema) or **serial testing to assess for stability** (e.g., serial H/H in a patient with a GI bleed).
- The patient **cannot tolerate P.O.** intake, has intractable **vomiting,** or has intractable **pain.**
- **Failure of outpatient management** with multiple bounce-back visits.
- **Social issues** like the patient cannot care for themselves at home due to the new illness and cannot realistically get to follow up.
- **The patient specifically requests admission** and doesn't feel safe going home.

In general, you should have a lower threshold to continue outpatient management if:

- None of the above admission criteria are met.
- The patient has a definitive diagnosis, and your clinical references show they meet the relevant set of "**Discharge criteria.**"
- The illness is **lower severity by risk calculators**
- They have **stable vital signs.**
- They are **ambulatory.**
- They are **tolerating P.O.** intake, and pain is controlled.
- The patient **feels comfortable and prefers going home.**

CONTINGENCY PLANNING WITH YOUR PATIENTS

You won't always get the diagnosis and disposition right. We all make mistakes from time to time, and that's okay. The important thing is to have a backup plan in the way of **good discharge instructions**. What should you advise your patients if they fail to improve after discharge?

Including **time-specific and action-specific** discharge instructions and **strict return precautions** are critical habits for safe medical practice. For example, "Please call to make an appointment with the gynecologist within the next two weeks to discuss your large left ovarian dermoid cyst. Please know that these cysts can twist and lose blood flow (i.e., ovarian torsion), which is a time-critical emergency. If you develop worsening pain, bleeding, vomiting, or lightheadedness, please go immediately to the emergency department."

One last technique to help you navigate grey-zone disposition situations is the **"pre-mortem analysis."** This involves you pausing to consider, "If I send my patient home and later find out they decompensated, what do I think would be the likely cause?" Instead of waiting for them to fail, this reflection attempts to predict and prevent it. When you discuss your hesitancy to send a patient home with your attending or specialist, you can verbalize specific concerns and explain why.

————

I hope these chapters have reinforced the concepts you learned in graduate school and explained exactly how you'll apply them to the patient in front of you. The importance of good clinical evaluation and reasoning cannot be overstated in the pursuit of practicing medicine safely. Next, we will dive deeper into interpreting all of the tests this section has helped us order.

CHAPTER 28
ACTION ITEMS

THE FOLLOWING action items can help you to evaluate patients, avoid forgetting assessments, and improve your diagnostic reasoning:

- Pause to determine whether your patient is an **"ABC or H&P patient."**
- Use a **systematic approach** for each patient, with a **checklist-style printout** if needed.
- Start making a **problem list** from the beginning of your interview.
- If you feel you are forgetting something, pause and consider the **prompt system**: Background-Foreground-DDx-Testing-Treatment-Disposition.
- Start a working **DDx** early in the case. For simple patient presentations, a brief **SPIT** DDx is often sufficient. For higher-risk patients, generate a longer DDx with an online **schema** (CP Solvers), **VINDICATE,** or **ChatGPT.**
- Favor **definitive** testing with high positive predictive value (PPV) and negative predictive value (NPV), as they will better help arrive at a final diagnosis.
- Medical decision-making starts with summarizing the key findings (**"signals"**) into a concise **problem statement** that informs the next steps.
- Practice this skill with the **"RLR CP Solvers"** podcast. Pause the podcast after each aliquot of information and express your thoughts.

- Consider **general admission criteria** like inability to eat/drink, ambulate, persistently abnormal vital signs, or failure of outpatient management for every patient.

Here are some **high-yield questions** to ask co-workers related to this section:

- How easy is it to transfer a decompensating patient out of our care? Are there any challenges or roadblocks to be aware of?
- Which are the most challenging/stressful patient presentations of our specialty?
- Do you have any pearls for sorting through these presentations?
- What medical decision-making errors do you see new grads making?
- How did you improve your assessment skills and critical thinking?

PART SIX
HOW TO INTERPRET TEST RESULTS

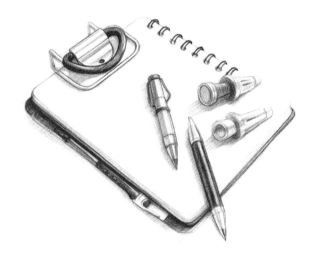

INTERPRETING DIAGNOSTIC TESTS

"I'm a new FNP, and I'm having a tough time interpreting test results and figuring out the next steps. I feel like my brain can't transfer what I knew from school tests to what I'm doing now. I also feel like school didn't differentiate the importance of some lab values over others. Any advice, resources, or tips to improve? Thanks in advance!"

FAMILY NURSE PRACTITIONER, 2023

Interpreting test results is a common area of stress for new graduates. The complexity is amplified in real-life patients who usually have more *abnormal* labs than *normal* ones. It's no wonder this aspect of clinical medicine causes heartburn for so many of us.

Four preparatory actions will help you better interpret lab results —

- **Re-learn the basics:** Go line by line down the lab reports where you work to ensure you know what each result means and how to interpret it. If you don't, review the fundamentals with an eye to actual clinical practice, not just passing a test. The Clinical Problem Solvers RLR website is a great place to do this. They share schemas for most abnormal labs and break things down into the essence of what you need to know.
- **Narrow your focus:** Search for your specialty's *top ten* most frequently ordered tests. Your review of lab core content should start with these.
- **Practice applying what you've learned**: The YouTube channel *Unremarkable Labs* does an excellent job presenting real patient cases with abnormal labs and encourages you to think critically about the next steps. Grow your skills with these high-yield cases.
- **Get the best on-shift references:** My favorite pocket reference is the "Clinician's Guide to Laboratory Medicine." This book has every lab result and a step-by-step action plan for each abnormality. Everything is clear and concise for reference while

at work. Ask your coworkers if they use any other lab references.

Once you start clinical practice, you'll notice a few test result patterns. First is the patient with a *single lab abnormality*, for whom algorithms can be beneficial in determining the next steps. Second is the patient with *multiple abnormalities*, for whom you'll have to consider whether one or multiple pathologies are causing the disturbances. Last is the situation with *all tests resulting normal*, which can also pose a unique challenge to the novice clinician. We will review all of these permutations in the following chapters.

Let's break down the most common diagnostic tests and how we interpret them in the real world:

- The complete blood count (CBC).
- The comprehensive metabolic panel (CMP).
- The blood gas (ABG and VBG).
- The electrocardiogram (ECG) .
- The approach to isolated abnormal test results.
- The approach to multiple abnormal test results.
- The approach to negative testing.

CHAPTER 29
DECODING THE CBC

Patient case: A 56-year-old female is brought for evaluation by her husband for constipation, abdominal cramping, chills, and fatigue. He thinks this is due to the chronically high doses of opioids she takes for back pain. An abdominal x-ray confirms a large amount of stool in the large intestine and rectum. A CBC notes a WBC of 11,000 with 30% bands. She improves with IV fluids, is diagnosed with constipation, and is discharged with a bowel regimen. Three days later, she returned with worsening symptoms and decompensated after having perforated stercoral colitis. Stercoral colitis is a complication of severe fecal impaction in which increased pressure causes a breakdown of the rectal mucosa.

THE CBC SEEMS like a simple test to interpret, but red flags can be buried on the lines toward the bottom. Dr. Chuck Pilcher is a medical malpractice expert who runs a free monthly newsletter and commented on the case above, "Overlooking bandemia happens all too often in patients who progress to sepsis, necrotizing fasciitis, perforated appendicitis, and more. Not addressing a sledgehammer like 30% bandemia is a major lapse. "[1]

---

1. Mad Mimi. "Archives: Medical Malpractice Insights." Accessed May 1, 2023. https://madmimi.com/p/5f4487.

This chapter will review the CBC, the key lines that can reflect subtle red flags, and offer frameworks for interpretation.

WBC	6.88	4.00 - 12.00 K/uL
RBC	5.22	4.00 - 5.50 mil/uL
Hgb	14.1	12.0 - 16.0 g/dL
Hct	43.0	37 - 47 %
MCV	82.4	80 - 98 fL
MCH	27.0	27 - 33 pg
MCHC	32.8	32 - 37 g/dL
RDW	12.8	11.5 - 15.0 %
Plt	263	150 - 450 K/uL
Differential type	Automated	
Abs neuts	4.40	1.80 - 7.80 K/uL
Abs immature grans	0.01	0.00 - 0.07 K/uL
Abs lymphs	1.89	0.80 - 3.30 K/uL
Abs monos	0.39	0.10 - 1.00 K/uL
Abs eos	0.16	0.00 - 0.40 K/uL
Abs basos	0.03	0.00 - 0.20 K/uL
Neuts	64.0	%
Immature grans	0.1	0.0 - 0.9 %
Lymphs	27.5	%
Monos	5.7	%
Eos	2.3	%
Basos	0.4	%

Example CBC result from my hospital. Do you know what every line means?

THE INITIAL APPROACH TO CBC INTERPRETATION

- What are the **"three cell lines"** of the CBC?
- How would you refer to a decrease in **all three** cell lines?

Think about the CBC as an assessment of the body's three cell lines: *red* blood cells (with Hgb), *white* blood cells (with their differential), and *platelets*.

When you see an abnormality in one cell line, **look to the other cell lines first.** You need to note if there are changes in multiple cell lines, such as a **pancytopenia** or a **bicytopenia**. A pancytopenia has a unique DDx and approach, considering serious issues like bone marrow failure.

140

Second, look for the **prior values to see if they are acute or chronic.**
Third, assess the patient for **symptoms** that would match the abnormality.
If they are asymptomatic, this will change management significantly.
After these initial steps, we dive into the specific approach for the most
common abnormalities.

———

THE ELEVATED WBC (LEUKOCYTOSIS)

Case practice: You are a family practice NP following up on lab results
for a 50-year-old female patient you recently saw for a routine physical
exam. They felt fine without acute complaints, yet their WBC is
elevated at 14,000. How do you proceed? Please also answer the
general questions below.

- What are the most common causes of a **moderately elevated**
  WBC of 12-20k?
- If there aren't any signs of infection, **what else should be
  considered on the DDx?**
- What must be added to the DDx when you note a **severely
  elevated** WBC of 30k and above?
- You've read that **"bands"** or **"bandemia"** (aka, a "left shift") is
  an ominous sign of a significant bacterial infection. Where can
  you find the band count on the initial CBC image?

If the **WBC is elevated,** the most common causes are infection and
inflammation. Faced with this, your job is to assess for a source of infection
and indicators for the severity of infection (e.g., SIRS and sepsis criteria).
However, if no infection is apparent, consider an expanded DDx for a
leukocytosis:

- **Occult bacteremia** (e.g., endocarditis, which often presents with
  subtle and nonspecific signs/symptoms. Inquire about risk
  factors like IVDU or dental procedures)
- **Inflammation** (e.g., autoimmune conditions like inflammatory
  bowel disease)

- **Medications** (e.g., corticosteroid use)
- **Smoking** and **illicit drug use**.
- If the WBC is sky high, add **heme-onc malignancies** (such as **leukemia**) to the DDx.
- **Stress demargination,** a term used to explain an elevated WBC in a state of physical or emotional stress. WBCs are thought to release from blood vessel walls in preparation for potential injury or infection. This is considered a diagnosis of exclusion.

Common new grad error: Ignoring the **differential**. Always review the differential to see which type of white blood cell is driving the change in the total WBC elevation. The DDx shared above reflects the most common situation of a "**neutrophil**-predominant leukocytosis." If you notice another type of white blood cell driving the change, the DDx and approach can change significantly:

- **Lymphocytosis**: High lymphocyte counts could be seen in certain viral infections like mononucleosis, pertussis, or lymphoproliferative disorders like chronic lymphocytic leukemia. Suspect mono if you notice a high *"reactive lymphocyte"* count.
- **Eosinophilia**: Eosinophil counts > 1500 can suggest allergic reactions (e.g., Drug reaction with eosinophilia and systemic symptoms (DRESS)), adrenal insufficiency, parasitic infections, or certain malignancies.
- **Blasts** and **elevated basophils** are both red flags for malignancy.

Common new grad error: Failing to recognize **bandemia**. Bands are often reported as *absolute immature granulocytes* on the differential. Bands >10% are a marker of severe bacterial infection, *even without an elevated WBC*. This is part of the SIRS criteria, which many clinicians forget.

Let's return to our patient case with routine lab testing noting a leukocytosis. Using what you've learned here, you first review the differential and confirm that the **neutrophil** count is elevated, driving the changes seen in the WBC. Your patient is asymptomatic, thus lowering the possibility of an infectious or inflammatory cause, and she hasn't taken any steroids recently. You consider the DDx and remember that the patient smokes cigarettes. You ask her to stop smoking and recheck the CBC after quitting, which normalizes.

THE LOW WBC (LEUKOPENIA)

- If the **WBC is low**, what should you look for next, and what is the highest-risk possibility?
- What are the causes of a low WBC?

If the WBC is low (*leukopenic*), scrutinize the differential and beware of the low neutrophil count (*neutropenic*).

Common new grad error: Failing to recognize the implications of neutropenia. Remember that our neutrophils are the immune system's main defense. **Neutropenic patients are considered potentially immunocompromised**, especially if the neutrophil count is under 500 (0.5 on the lab's reference range above), which is severe range neutropenia.

Relatively benign causes of a low WBC include familial/genetic causes (in which case the patient would be chronically leukopenic/neutropenic and not immunocompromised) and viral infections. Dangerous causes of a low WBC include bone marrow failure, immunosuppressive medications (e.g., chemotherapy), or overwhelming infections. Regardless of the cause, we must take infectious complaints more seriously in these patients.

––––––

THE LOW HGB (ANEMIA)

Case practice: You are an urgent care PA with on-site testing available. Your patient is a 54-year-old male presenting with fatigue over the past week. You order blood tests with the CBC demonstrating a new anemia with a hemoglobin of 10g/dL and a normal MCV. His prior values demonstrate a Hgb of 14g/dL two months ago. How would you approach the workup of this patient? Please also answer the general questions below.

- If the Hgb is low, what should you look for next on the CBC to better characterize the anemia and narrow the DDx?

- What are three causes of acute anemias?
- What Hgb level is considered severe and necessitates transfusion?

Anemia is *the most common* CBC abnormality you'll encounter in practice. Typically, this is a chronic and unsurprising anemia based on the patient's PMHx.

Here are a few common and expected anemia scenarios:

- **A female of childbearing age with heavy menstrual periods and a chronic microcytic anemia:** This is iron deficiency anemia from blood loss, you should advise her to take iron supplements and recheck her CBC to ensure it normalizes.
- **An adult with severe alcohol use disorder and chronic malnutrition with a chronic macrocytic anemia:** This is related to nutritional deficiencies like B12, folate, and alcohol use. Advise cessation, recommend multivitamins, and periodically recheck to ensure improvement.
- **An adult with advanced organ disease (kidney disease, liver disease, etc) and a chronic normocytic anemia:** This is anemia of chronic disease, the underlying disease should be treated, and outpatient specialties can consider other treatment modalities to improve the anemia.

Common new grad error: Becoming accustomed to seeing anemias daily and letting down their guard for serious causes. When is low hemoglobin **a red flag for a dangerous situation?**

The first red flag is **chronic anemia** *in a patient with no reason for it.* Consider the 60-year-old male with no PMHx and a gradually worsening microcytic anemia who denies external bleeding. This is not a patient you would expect to see anemia. You must consider the possibility of a malignancy like colon cancer with chronic GI bleeding.

The second red flag is **any severe anemia.** A Hgb **below 7 g/dL** is considered severe and requires transfusion.

The third red flag is **any *acute* anemia.** You'll be lucky to have prior labs to confirm an acute change in the labs. If you don't have recent labs, consider acute anemia if your patient has a *recent onset of symptoms plus anemia with a normal MCV.* The normal MCV might suggest there hasn't been enough time for compensation. This is what occurred in our anemia patient's vignette above.

Here are three important causes of *acute* anemias —

- **Bleeding**: Ask about external bleeding, bloody stools, black tarry stools, or recent trauma.
- **Hemolysis:** Consider this high-risk condition whenever you note the pattern of *anemia + elevated bilirubin +/- elevated AST*. Look for other markers of hemolysis like *low haptoglobin,* as well as *low platelets.*
- **Bone marrow failure:** Consider this high-risk condition whenever you note a *pancytopenia* or a *low reticulocyte count.*

Check out the great algorithms shared by the Manual of Medicine for evaluating anemia and the DDx by Dr. Khudhur Moh.[2,3]

THE LOW PLATELET COUNT (THROMBOCYTOPENIA)

- What are the risks of low platelets?
- What are the most common causes, and "can't miss" causes of thrombocytopenia?
- How would you evaluate a patient with thrombocytopenia to determine the cause?

If you see **low platelets**, recognize that the severity correlates with the bleeding risk. The bleeding risk increases when platelets drop below *50,000*. Platelets under *20,000* significantly increase the risk of spontaneous bleeding.

2. Shade191. "Anemia: Approach and Evaluation." *Manual of Medicine* (blog), January 3, 2022. https://manualofmedicine.com/topics/hematology-oncology/anemia-approach-and-evaluation/.
3. https://x.com/khudhur_moh/status/1444323338818625549

Always try to find the cause of the low platelets. There are three "can't miss" causes of thrombocytopenia to consider:

- **Platelet production problems:** In conditions like aplastic anemia, HIV, and leukemia, bone marrow failure results in decreased production of platelets as well as the other cell lines. Consider these possibilities whenever you note pancytopenia or other features of HIV/leukemia.
- **Platelet destruction problems:** In autoimmune conditions like immune thrombocytopenic purpura (ITP), antibodies target platelets resulting in destruction and significantly low platelet counts. Platelet counts can become severely low, increasing bleeding risk.
- **Platelet consumption problems:** In the family of conditions referred to as thrombotic microangiopathies (TMA) or microangiopathic hemolytic anemias (MAHA), a systemic illness like DIC or TTP results in platelet clumping in small blood vessels. As a result, RBCs are sheared as they pass through these vessels, causing hemolysis. MAHA disorders are all considered very high risk. The lab pattern to recognize these disorders is anemia, thrombocytopenia, elevated bilirubin, and AST elevation. *Heparin-induced thrombocytopenia (HIT)* is another life-threatening condition in which patients who received heparin (even a heparin flush!) can have an immune-mediated response causing hypercoagulability despite seeing low platelet counts on labs. Consider this possibility whenever you note decreasing platelet levels or inappropriate clotting in a patient who received heparin.

Here is one step-wise approach to evaluating thrombocytopenia shared by the Curbsiders that incorporates dangerous causes as well as common causes:

- Is the thrombocytopenia isolated or accompanied by anemia and leukopenia?
- Review the patient's medication list and note any recent changes or exposures (e.g., antibiotics, chemotherapy, anti-depressants).
- Is there evidence of hemolysis? (Anemia, thrombocytopenia, elevated bilirubin, and AST elevation).

- Consider DIC, TTP/HUS, HIT or acute leukemia in patients who look sick.
- Ask about hepatitis C, HIV, and if dyspepsia is present, H. pylori infection.
- Determine if the patient is at risk for nutritional deficiencies.
- Do they have known liver disease (hypersplenism from portal hypertension or decreased production of thrombopoietin), thyroid disease, autoimmune or rheumatologic conditions?

Check out one of Dr. Matt Ho's Twitter algorithms that share an algorithm for working this up.[4] Dr. Khudhur Moh has another figure summarizing his approach to thrombocytopenia here:

4. Matthew Ho, MD PhD [@MatthewHoMD]. "Consolidated Flowcharts on 1. Approach to Bleeding 2. Working up Thrombocytopenia 3. Working up Elevated PT and/or APTT 4. Working up VWD Https://T.Co/JkRVJb1x9V." Tweet. *Twitter*, February 4, 2023. https://twitter.com/MatthewHoMD/status/1621881585199976452.

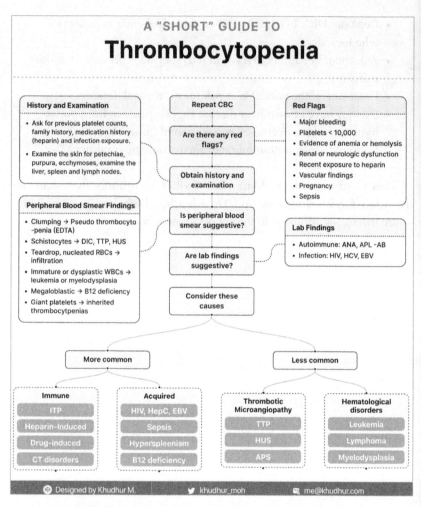

Dr. Khudhur Moh's approach to thrombocytopenia, with permission

If you struggle interpreting the CBC, solidify your knowledge by listening to the fantastic Curbsider's podcast episode 167, dedicated entirely to CBC interpretation. One last pearl Dr. Mary Kwok MD shared on the Curbsiders episode: "Repeat the CBC before referring patients to hematology." Sometimes things like platelet clumping can lead to falsely abnormal blood tests.

In review, respect the highest-risk lab results on the CBC:

- **Pancytopenia** or **anemia plus a low reticulocyte count**: Both suggest bone marrow failure.
- **Bandemia**: >10% suggests a severe bacterial infection.
- **Neutropenia**: Especially if under 500 neutrophils (0.5 on most labs), potentially suggesting an immunocompromised state.
- **Thrombocytopenia**: Severe range and bleeding risk occur under 50k, but all acute thrombocytopenias should have the dangerous causes excluded.
- **Hgb under 7**, or an **acute drop in Hgb:** Consider the three dangerous causes of acute anemia (bleeding, hemolysis, production failure).
- The pattern of **anemia + elevated bilirubin, AST, +/- thrombocytopenia:** Consider hemolysis and MAHA disorders.

CHAPTER 30
DISSECTING THE CMP

Na	136	135 - 145 mmol/L
K	4.1	3.6 - 5.3 mmol/L
Cl	103	98 - 109 mmol/L
CO2	22	21 - 32 mmol/L
Anion gap w/o K	11	7 - 15
BUN	8	8 - 24 mg/dL
Creatinine	0.96	0.6 - 1.2 mg/dL
GFR non African Amer	62	>59 mL/min
GFR African American	75	>59 mL/min
Glucose	104	65 - 120 mg/dL
SGOT/AST	14	5 - 40 IU/L
Alk Phos	55	28 - 126 IU/L
SGPT/ALT	12	6 - 60 IU/L
Bilirubin total	0.5	0.2 - 1.4 mg/dL
Protein	6.7	6.2 - 8.0 g/dL
Albumin	3.8	3.2 - 5.0 g/dL
Globulin (calc)	2.9	2.0 - 4.5 g/dL
A:G Ratio	1.3	>1.0
Calcium	9.1	8.5 - 10.5 mg/dL

Example CMP result from my hospital

THE METABOLIC PANEL is more complex than meets the eye. You could easily find three hours of lectures for each line of the CMP. Respect the internist's depth of knowledge! Let's break down the most important aspects of the metabolic panel.

SODIUM DERANGEMENTS

Case practice: You are a hospitalist NP sent to admit a patient from the ED. The patient is 82 years old and was brought to the hospital by their family for a one-week history of fatigue, generalized weakness, and lack of appetite. The ED found the patient hyponatremic to 122 mEq/L (reference range 135-145). How would you evaluate and manage this patient? Please also answer the questions below.

- What is your approach to **hyponatremia**?
- And **hypernatremia**?
- How should you correct sodium abnormalities?

The sodium (Na) level on the BMP is a function of *volume and water balance* and typically does *not* reflect a sodium intake problem. So, when you see low sodium, don't assume it's because the patient isn't taking in enough salt. It's much more likely that their body isn't excreting free water, leading to a dilutional effect on the serum sodium.

Hyponatremia is one of the most common electrolyte abnormalities encountered in hospitalized patients. Your first step should be to look at the glucose, since hyperglycemia can cause "pseudo-hyponatremia" that you won't have to worry about. If it is true hyponatremia, try categorizing the sodium changes as *acute or chronic* and *symptomatic or asymptomatic*. Hyponatremia is the highest risk and requires immediate treatment if the patient is seizing, altered, or with focal deficits. The severe range of sodium is under 120. However, even a mild hyponatremia of 130 deserves a plan to assess and fix it. The key is to fix it slowly in most patients.

Common new grad error: Correcting an abnormal sodium too quickly in chronic or asymptomatic patients, putting them at risk of osmotic demyelination or cerebral edema. Most patients should have their hyponatremia raised by **4-6 mEq/L in a 24-hour period.** This is easy to overshoot even with normal saline. Hypertonic saline and free water are *high-risk medications* that should only be ordered in consultation with your attending.

Narrowing down the cause of hyponatremia is reviewed in Dr. Moh's hyponatremia approach algorithm below. Conceptually, hyponatremia typically occurs when the kidneys stop excreting free water, resulting in a dilution of sodium in the blood. The kidneys most commonly stop excreting free water when anti-diuretic hormone (ADH) is turned on, which can occur for many reasons like pain, nausea, dehydration, poor cardiac output/perfusion, cancer, drugs, and more. If there isn't a physiologic stimulus for ADH being turned on, you might be dealing with the "syndrome of inappropriate ADH" (SIADH).

Perhaps the most dangerous underlying etiology to always consider whenever you see low sodium is **adrenal insufficiency or adrenal crisis**, as these patients can quickly decompensate if left untreated. Pause to assess for other features that might suggest this possibility:

- Elevated potassium.
- Low blood sugar.
- Low blood pressure or temperature.
- Elevated eosinophil count.
- Chronic steroid use plus dosing decrease or infection/trauma.
- Tan skin, as seen in primary adrenal insufficiency (i.e., Addison's disease).

For more information, check out the best hyponatremia reviews: CoreIM has a fantastic two-part podcast series, and the Curbsiders invited nephrologist Joel Topf for dedicated episodes on hyponatremia and hypernatremia. The next page shares another of Dr. Mo's fantastic algorithms.[1]

---

1. https://x.com/khudhur_moh/status/1564311500852023297

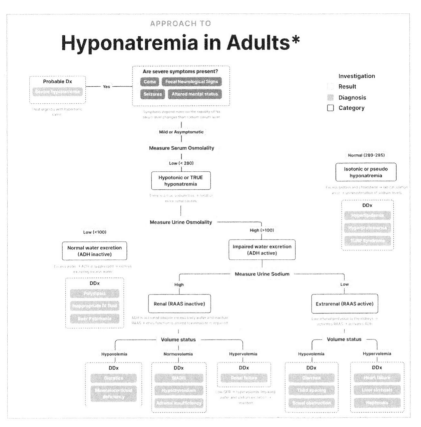

Khudhur Mo, with permission. Download the high-resolution PDF at the footnote on the prior page.

POTASSIUM DERANGEMENTS

- What is your approach to **hyperkalemia** (the most dangerous electrolyte abnormality)?
- What are the risks and the most important next steps if it is true hyperkalemia?
- What is your approach to **hypokalemia**?
- What are the risks of hypokalemia, and what other lab should be checked?
- What **EKG changes** would you expect with each?

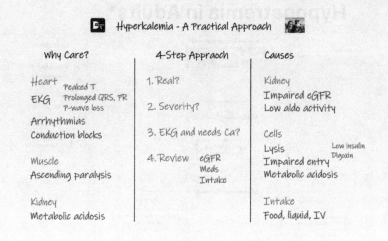

Why Care?	4-Step Approach	Causes
Heart	1. Real?	Kidney
Peaked T		Impaired eGFR
EKG Prolonged QRS, PR		Low aldo activity
P-wave loss	2. Severity?	
Arrhythmias		Cells
Conduction blocks	3. EKG and needs Ca?	Lysis Low insulin
		Impaired entry Digoxin
Muscle	4. Review eGFR	Metabolic acidosis
Ascending paralysis	Meds	
	Intake	
Kidney		Intake
Metabolic acidosis		Food, liquid, IV

CP Solvers hyperkalemia approach, with permission

Think of **potassium (K) as the "heart's electrolyte."** With a significantly deranged K, the first step is to look for evidence of "pseudo-hyperkalemia" (**hemolysis** during lab draw, which the lab can clarify). If hemolysis is ruled out, outpatient providers should refer these patients to the ED, given how dangerous it can be.

The second step is to get an **EKG**. Two memory aids will help you remember the EKG changes with potassium derangements. First, think **"potassium lives in the T waves:"** With high potassium, you'll see big peaked T waves, and with low potassium, you'll see flat or inverted T waves. Remember the other EKG changes of hyperkalemia by imagining a **fisherman snagging a T wave, pulling up and to the right**. First, you'll see the peaked T waves, then you'll see a widened PR and QRS. Last, remember that **hyperkalemia can cause bradycardia and heart blocks.**

Even at the beginning of a patient encounter, if you see a newly wide-complex EKG that looks like VTach but has a *slow rate*, this is a fairly unique finding suggesting hyperkalemia. I'll share an example of this in the EKG chapters coming up soon.

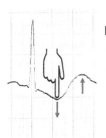

Hypokalaemia

T wave inversion
ST depression
Prominent U wave

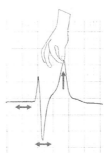

Hyperkalaemia

Peaked T waves
P wave flattening
PR prolongation
Wide QRS complex

Common new grad error: Not appreciating the risk of hyperkalemia. **Hyperkalemia with EKG changes is life-threatening and must be immediately managed.**

A rule of thumb is anything over **6.5** is the highest risk. However, any degree of hyperkalemia can put the patient at risk of dysrhythmias (especially if it's an acute rise).[2] All hyperkalemia should have a plan to fix it, even if mild and without EKG changes. Hyperkalemia is very common, typically seen in patients with ESRD, so you need to know this topic well.

Check a magnesium level whenever you see **hypokalemia**, as you won't be able to correct hypokalemia until the magnesium level is normalized. One example algorithm shared by a major nephrology association in the United Kingdom is on the next page. Learn more at the excellent summary here: https://emcrit.org/ibcc/hyperkalemia/

---

2. Simon LV, Hashmi MF, Farrell MW. Hyperkalemia. [Updated 2023 Feb 19]. In: StatPearls [Internet]. Treasure Island (FL): StatPearls Publishing; 2023 Jan-. Available from: https://www.ncbi.nlm.nih.gov/books/NBK470284/

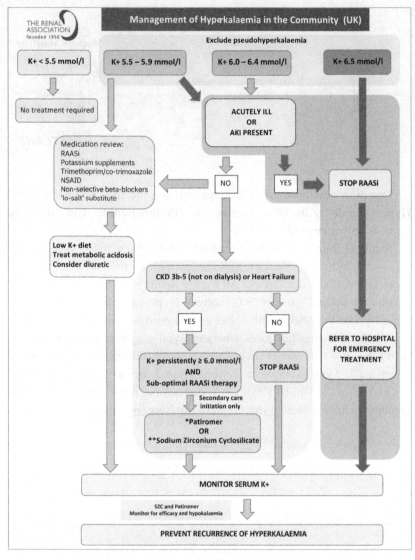

The United Kingdom's Kidney Association 2020 Hyperkalemia Guidelines

CHLORIDE LEVELS

- What lab changes would you expect when giving someone multiple liters of normal saline (a "hyperchloremic solution")?

Chloride (Cl) levels can be easy to overlook. Chloride is the primary anion in the extracellular space and is the counterpart to the main cation, sodium. Thus, Cl level changes typically reflect changes in serum sodium. A low Cl is also seen in nausea and vomiting (HCl loss). If the Cl is low from significant vomiting, giving them a hyperchloremic solution like normal saline makes good physiologic sense.

Common new grad error: Giving multiple liters of normal saline to a patient with normal electrolytes, therefore causing an acidosis. Giving large volumes of normal saline (NaCl) packed full of chloride to a patient with a normal chloride level will push bicarbonate out due to the net neutrality of anions. This loss of bicarb causes a non-anion gap metabolic acidosis. Thus, many prefer a balanced solution like **lactated ringers (LR)** for a more normal electrolyte profile during large-volume fluid resuscitation that won't result in acidosis.

CO2 AND THE ANION GAP

- What does the "CO2" refer to when listed on the metabolic panel?
- What does the "CO2" refer to when listed on blood gas results?

Bicarbonate (listed as CO2 on the metabolic panel) and the anion gap is your window into the patient's acid-base status without needing a dedicated blood gas. A high or low bicarb cannot be ignored. Acid-base problems will be covered in the next chapter.

———

BUN AND CREATININE

Case practice: You are an EM PA caring for a 75-year-old male with a PMHx of DM2 who presents to the ED reporting fevers, productive cough, and fatigue. The workup notes an elevated WBC, a creatinine of 2.0mg/dL (baseline 1.0), BUN of 42 mg/dL, and a potassium of 5.2 mEq/L. What could be the cause, and how would you treat his AKI? Please also answer the questions below.

- If you notice a newly elevated creatinine, how can you classify the type of acute kidney injury?
- What is the expected BUN: Creatinine ratio for the most common situation of a pre-renal AKI?
- What else might cause an elevated BUN?

Remember the **ratio of BUN to creatinine** can help further delineate the cause of an acute kidney injury. A high BUN with only mild to moderately elevated creatinine, as seen on a BUN:Creat ratio over 20, suggests a pre-renal AKI. Functional excretion of Na (FeNa) can also be calculated to help narrow the cause.

Pre-renal AKIs are the most common and reflect a problem in the rest of the body that results in poorer kidney perfusion — often from dehydration or hypotension. In the case above, it might be malperfusion from sepsis.

Per Dr. Joel Topf, **you can fix 90% of AKIs by doing three things:**

- **Giving fluids** (addressing most pre-renal causes like dehydration).
- **Avoiding nephrotoxins** (addressing most intra-renal treatments which involve supportive care).
- **Checking a bladder scan** and putting in a Foley catheter if there is urinary retention (addressing post-renal causes).

Check out Dr. Topf's great Curbsiders AKI podcast episode. This article shares an excellent algorithm to work up AKIs.[3] **Last pearl:** Remember that BUN changes can occur from multiple causes beyond acute kidney injuries. BUN can be low in malnourished patients and elevated in patients with GI bleeds. When upper GI bleeding occurs, the blood is digested into protein, absorbed, and metabolized into BUN.

––––––

3. Mo, Sophy. "Approach to Acute Kidney Injury." *McGill Journal of Medicine* 20, no. 2 (April 19, 2022). https://doi.org/10.26443/mjm.v20i2.943.

LIVER TESTS

- How would you classify a patient's abnormal liver tests into the buckets of "**hepatocellular** or **cholestatic**" injury patterns?
- Are "liver function tests" (LFTs) actual tests of liver function? If not, what tests truly demonstrate whether or not a patient's liver is functioning well?
- If you notice a significantly elevated AST without other liver test abnormalities, what could this be from?

Common new grad error: Thinking LFTs are specific to the liver and its function.

"Liver function tests" (LFTs: AST, ALT) are NOT tests of liver function, but rather intracellular enzymes frequently seen in liver disease or injury. AST, however, is much less specific to the liver and is inside many cells around the body. Thus, if you see an isolated sky-high AST and otherwise normal LFTs, think of something else like rhabdomyolysis or hemolysis.

The liver's *function* is to synthesize specific proteins and clear bilirubin. Suppose a hepatologist asks about your patient's liver function. They are referring to things like *INR* (liver failure results in high INR), *bilirubin* (high bilirubin), *platelet count* (low platelets), and *albumin* (low albumin).

Alkaline phosphatase and bilirubin comprise the additional components necessary to categorize liver injuries as hepatocellular versus cholestatic injury patterns that help narrow the cause. A severely elevated AST/ALT with mild to moderately elevated alk phos and bilirubin suggests a hepatocellular pattern of injury (e.g., viral hepatitis, drug-induced liver injury from acetaminophen, autoimmune, ischemic, or alcoholic hepatitis). A significantly elevated alk phos and bilirubin elevation with mild AST/ALT elevation suggests a cholestatic injury pattern (i.e., blockage of the bile ducts by stones, tumors, or other infiltrative processes).

Be mindful that alk phos is nonspecific and can be elevated in other conditions like bone disease and cancer. GGT is sometimes used to help clarify whether there is a biliary disturbance, but even GGT is nonspecific and can be elevated for other reasons.

Dr. Elliot Tapper is a famous hepatologist (@ebtapper on Twitter) who shared a great pearl on the Curbsiders episode 293, "In patients with LFT derangements, pay particular attention to the bilirubin. The bilirubin is the thermometer for disease severity across multiple liver pathologies. The higher the bilirubin, the more afraid I get and the lower my threshold to admit the patient."

For further reading, here is another great algorithm for working up abnormal LFTs.[4]

CALCIUM LEVELS

- If you see abnormalities in the calcium level on a metabolic panel, what should you next check on the metabolic panel?
- What conditions should you consider if the patient has true hypercalcemia or hypocalcemia?

Calcium (Ca) on a metabolic panel refers to total calcium, including the calcium bound to albumin. It does not reflect the level of calcium the body physiologically "feels" from the *ionized* calcium. The albumin level will heavily influence the Ca level on the BMP. If you notice a low Ca level, look at the albumin level and consider ordering an *ionized* calcium level. When the patient is hypercalcemic, the most common causes include ingestions (drugs and milk-alkali syndrome), malignancy, and endocrinopathies (PTH derangements).

Check out the Clinical Problem Solvers hypercalcemia schema.[5] For a deeper dive into the causes and treatment of hypercalcemia, check out this detailed discussion by the Curbsiders: https://thecurbsiders.com/podcast/281.

In review, respect the highest-risk lab results on the CMP —

- **Hyponatremia**: Under **120** is severe, and under **130** is moderate. Always consider adrenal insufficiency and avoid rapid correction outside the few indications noted above.

4. Zhuoer (Zoey) Xie, MD, MSCR [@ZhuoerXie]. "Algorithm for LFT Workup #MedTwitter Https://T.Co/YfvlJQYeGm." Tweet. *Twitter*, March 18, 2023. https://twitter.com/ZhuoerXie/status/1637205298757640192.
5. https://clinicalproblemsolving.com/dx-schema-hypercalcemia/

- **Hyperkalemia**: A rule of thumb is anything over **6.5** is the highest risk. However, any degree of hyperkalemia can put the patient at risk of dysrhythmias (especially if it's an acute rise).[6]
- **Low bicarbonate:** Under **12** is severe, and under **16** is moderate. All decreased bicarbonate levels warrant an explanation.
- **Elevated bilirubin:** Over **3** is considered moderately elevated, but all elevated bilirubin warrants a DDx consideration. The higher the bilirubin, the lower the threshold to admit the patient.
- **Hypercalcemia** (severe if over 14) or **hypocalcemia** (severe if under 7).

6. Simon LV, Hashmi MF, Farrell MW. Hyperkalemia. [Updated 2023 Feb 19]. In: StatPearls [Internet]. Treasure Island (FL): StatPearls Publishing; 2023 Jan-. Available from: https://www.ncbi.nlm.nih.gov/books/NBK470284/

CHAPTER 31

A SIMPLIFIED APPROACH TO ACID-BASE

ENTER another topic feared by most new graduates: acid-base. The depth of knowledge you'll need will depend upon your specialty, with critical care requiring the most robust understanding. However, even if you aren't in the ICU, every specialty needs to know the basics.

The goal of evaluating acid-base problems is indirect. We don't identify an acidosis and react by giving bicarbonate. Our goal is to identify an acidosis, *seek out the underlying cause*, and treat that cause.

For instance, if a pregnant woman with hyperemesis gravidarum has an acidosis due to ketone production in her starving state, we treat her with anti-nausea medications, give her carbohydrates, and the body takes care of the acid-base problem on its own. We will see this concept echoed in all the case studies below.

Graduate school often teaches acid-base in a way that doesn't usually come up in clinical practice, which is part of why I think this is a tricky topic for so many. Graduate school teaches the relevant players that determine the acid-base status:

- **pH**, or the net acidity of the blood.
- **pCO2**, or carbon dioxide
- **Bicarbonate**. Labs list the bicarbonate as *CO2* on a BMP and as *HCO3* on a blood gas.
- **The anion gap**, which is the difference between the anions and cations, the electrolytes reported in our BMP

Many new grads get confused when they see "CO2" on a metabolic panel and think this refers to carbon dioxide. Remember, the CO2 listed on the metabolic panel is the **bicarbonate** — a historical labeling convention.

Another common source of confusion is the many equations we're taught to use. However, many of these equations aren't necessary for common scenarios in well-appearing patients. The equations should be learned eventually if you manage sick patients. To memorize these formulas, I recommend Joel Topf's podcast on acid-base and the acid-base overview post in EMCrit's Internet Book of Critical Care. Both provide a digestible summary of these topics.

For now, I want to make sure you can identify that you are dealing with an "acid-base patient" and know the first few steps clinicians take.

Statistically speaking, you are most likely to encounter a metabolic acidosis. How do these manifest? It all starts with the results on the metabolic panel.

CASE ONE

A 32-year-old insulin-dependent diabetic patient presents with abdominal pain and nausea. The metabolic panel reveals:

- **Na: 132** (Normal range: 135 - 145)
- **K: 5.3** (3.6 - 5.3)
- **Cl: 96** (98 - 109)
- **CO2: 16** (21-32)
- **AG = 20** [Calculation: Na 132 - (Cl 96+ bicarb 16) = 20]
- **BUN: 24** (8 - 24)
- **Creatinine: 0.95** (0.6-1.2)
- **Glucose: >599**

Our first clue to an acid-base problem is the **low bicarbonate (CO2) level**. When you see *low bicarb*, think *metabolic acidosis*, and you'll be right 99% of the time. You technically can't confirm it is a metabolic acidosis without running a dedicated blood gas, but exceptions to this rule of thumb are rare for ambulatory patients outside the ICU.

After identifying an acidosis, the next question is, *"What is the anion gap?"* In this case, it is elevated. This helps refine our clinical picture to a **high anion gap metabolic acidosis (HAGMA)**, which narrows the DDx. You were likely taught the DDx MUDPILES, a comprehensive list with things like paraldehyde you'll never see. I was taught that **KULT** (a shortened form of MUDPILES) is easier to remember and will identify 95+% of the causes of HAGMAs.

1. **K** = **ketone** production, as is seen in DKA (diabetic ketoacidosis), AKA (alcoholic ketoacidosis), or starvation ketosis like in our hyperemesis patient earlier. The blood sugar levels or the overall clinical picture will suggest these possibilities. If your patient says they are on a "keto diet," that's another clear giveaway!
2. **U** = **uremia** or renal failure with high BUN, high creatinine, and low GFR (resulting in accumulation of phosphates and sulfates causing the acidosis).
3. **L** = **lactate** elevation. You can order a serum lactate level when it makes sense clinically, like in sepsis or the elderly patient with acute severe abdominal pain from mesenteric ischemia resulting in lactic acidosis. Remember there are many other causes of lactate elevation.[1]
4. **T** = **toxins.** Ask the patient if they drank alcohol or another intoxicating substance. Ask if they've been taking any medication recently, like aspirin or acetaminophen. Ask if they are suicidal. If any are positive, send a serum ASA/APAP level and serum osmolality to assess for an osmolar gap, which would highly suggest toxic alcohol ingestion (e.g., ethylene glycol or methanol).

Each of these four conditions involves *the addition of* an acidic substance that drops the bicarbonate via buffering and displaces the body's normal anions. This anion displacement is why these four conditions cause a "widened anion gap." Contrast this with the *normal anion gap* NAGMAs below, which don't *add* an acidic substance but rather simply *lose* bicarbonate. Direct bicarbonate loss doesn't displace any anions, so the anion gap remains normal in those conditions.

It should then make sense why an attending might ask you, "What *substance* do you think is driving the widened anion gap?" With the provided case example, we can immediately sort out the acid-base problem without needing a blood gas analysis. After noting the HAGMA, we can review the KULT DDx to see if any of the possibilities fit. This

---

1. The Clinical Problem Solvers. "Dx Schema – Lactic Acidosis," March 11, 2020. https://clinicalproblemsolving.com/dx-schema-lactic-acidosis/.

patient is diabetic with uncontrolled hyperglycemia, so our suspected cause is ketones from a mild DKA/insulin-deficient state. We then ask the patient if they've been taking their insulin. They respond, "I might have run out of my insulin a week ago." Clinical diagnosis made.

Some clinicians might send confirmatory testing for ketones like beta-hydroxybutyrate or a VBG. However, many won't bother, because getting a dedicated blood gas in this case probably won't change management. These are often deferred if the clinical picture is clear and the derangements aren't severe. We can treat the patient by giving fluids and insulin to get them out of ketosis and recheck a metabolic panel to ensure resolution.

If you can't find the cause of the HAGMA after reviewing KULT, do a web search for "MUDPILES" and dive deeper through this DDx. In my opinion, memorizing MUDPILES early in your career is limited in utility when you can look it up as needed.

CASE TWO

The second situation to recognize is the **non-anion gap metabolic acidosis (NAGMA)**, which also has a unique DDx. Consider this example case: a 40-year-old patient presents with severe diarrhea persisting for two weeks. Their metabolic panel reveals the following:

- **Na: 136** (Normal range: 135 - 145)
- **K: 3.4** (3.6 - 5.3)
- **Cl: 112** (98 - 109)
- **CO2: 15** (21-32)
- **AG = 9** [Calculation: Na 136 - (Cl 112 + bicarb 15) = 9]
- **BUN: 30** (8 - 24)
- **Creatinine: 1.5** (0.6-1.2)
- **Glucose: >105**

Again, we notice a low bicarb, suggesting metabolic acidosis, but the anion gap is normal this time, giving us a NAGMA. **NAGMAs have a short list of potential causes that all directly drop the bicarbonate:**

1. **GI losses of bicarbonate-rich fluid** (diarrhea, ileostomy, etc.).
2. **Renal pathologies that inhibit the kidney's ability to retain bicarb,** as seen in renal insufficiency and renal tubular acidosis (RTA).

3. **Medications that induce renal losses of bicarb,** like acetazolamide.
4. **Large volumes of normal saline that result in high chloride levels.** High chloride (a negatively charged anion) then forces bicarbonate (also negatively charged) to move intracellularly to maintain ion equilibrium. This reduces the available bicarbonate and causes acidosis.
5. **Ureteral diversions that lower bicarbonate levels.** These are post-surgical and should be chronic.

In our case, the patient was not given normal saline, there were no signs of renal insufficiency, and the profuse diarrhea was the evident source of bicarbonate loss. Our working diagnosis is promptly made, and treatment focuses on addressing the underlying cause. The metabolic panel is then rechecked to ensure resolution. Note that most patients with diarrhea will not have associated acidosis. The presence of acidosis in our patient underscores the severity of his symptoms.

METABOLIC ALKALOSIS

Metabolic alkalosis is not quite as common. An increase in pH from a primary **increase** in bicarbonate concentration defines it. This condition can occur due to *a loss of hydrogen ions* (e.g., **losing stomach acid through vomiting,** or **diuretic therapy**) or *a gain in bicarbonate ions* as in the following situations:

1. **Alkaline drug administration**, like antacids.
2. **Volume loss** with the kidneys' response resulting in **increased bicarbonate concentration** (i.e., a "contraction alkalosis").
3. **Excess aldosterone/mineralocorticoid activity or steroid use.**

Remember the classic boards question: What is the expected electrolyte derangement after profuse vomiting? Answer: Hypokalemic hypochloremic metabolic alkalosis. Managing metabolic alkalosis involves treating the underlying cause, such as discontinuing the offending drug or treating the underlying illness.

Whenever you notice an elevated bicarbonate level on a metabolic panel, before assuming it is metabolic alkalosis, pause to consider whether it is compensation for a respiratory problem like COPD or obesity hypoventilation syndrome. In these cases, the high bicarb (a base) is the body's way of balancing out the high pCO2 (an acid) from these lung diseases.

The clinical picture will often suggest whether there is a respiratory problem (e.g., COPD) or if there is a metabolic problem (e.g., vomiting) driving the high bicarb. Regardless, you should still order a venous blood gas to confirm your suspicion by detailing the pH and pCO2 levels. A low pH and high pCO2 confirm a primary respiratory acidosis, and a high pH and a high bicarb confirm a primary metabolic alkalosis.

RESPIRATORY CASES

Respiratory acidosis and **respiratory alkalosis** tend to come more into the picture with (you guessed it) respiratory conditions, which are often apparent clinically. Your sick COPD patients, asthmatics, or vented patients will all have unique acid-base profiles that are usually straightforward to interpret.

As discussed, your COPD patient will generally have a high pCO2 as they are chronic pCO2 retainers. You can see how well they are compensating by looking at their pH and bicarb on an ABG. If their bicarb is high with a near-normal pH, then they are compensating well. However, if their pH is low, that is a bad sign of failure to compensate and indicates they need more support (in the form of BiPAP and other COPD treatments).

Trending ABGs in this situation can give helpful objective data trends in your higher-risk patients. Over time, you can learn the equations to calculate the expected values for acute versus chronic respiratory conditions, with or without compensation, and A-a gradient calculations. First, I'd encourage you to develop a conceptual understanding of what is being reflected in the blood gas results.

ORDERING BLOOD GASSES...

We've discussed how some common, mild acid-base derangements might not require a dedicated blood gas to develop a treatment plan. However, **when do you need to get a dedicated blood gas?**

1. If your **bicarbonate is elevated**, you'll want to verify the pH and pCO2 to determine whether it's driven by a respiratory or metabolic process.

2. If your **bicarbonate is moderate to severely low,** a blood gas will verify the severity of the situation via the pH. A pH under 7.1 directly reflects a critically ill patient, whereas a low bicarbonate only suggests the severity.
3. If you note a **significantly elevated anion gap with a normal bicarbonate**, this can suggest a mixed acid-base process that mandates further workup.
4. If you **need to know the exact PaO2**, to calculate an A-a gradient or titrate vent settings. This is commonly needed in intubated patients or those in whom the pulse oximeter is not giving reliable readings (e.g., cardiogenic shock).
5. If you're **unsure of the diagnosis** based on the metabolic panel and the clinical picture, getting a dedicated blood gas and performing the calculations can help narrow the DDx.

If you decide you need a blood gas, the question often arises: "When do I need an **arterial** blood gas (which is more invasive, more painful, and harder to get), and when can I use a **venous** blood gas instead?"

The historic gold standard for all acid-base evaluation has been an ABG, but in recent years studies have shown that the VBG will give accurate enough results for the pH and pCO2 to act on clinically. As a result, **if you are only concerned about a metabolic process, a VBG is usually fine.** If you are worried about **a respiratory problem** and want the true oxygen state (PaO2) to calculate an A-a gradient, then an **ABG is recommended.**

This chapter reviewed the absolute basics and left out some important situations like mixed acid-base issues. Read the Internet Book of Critical Care acid-base chapters for a deeper dive. They share a step-by-step acid-base approach incorporating the calculations you've likely been exposed to in graduate school. For fantastic practice cases, check out these websites:

- https://ABG.ninja
- http://www.meddean.luc.edu/lumen/med-ed/mech/cases/case26/Caseqa_f.htm

CHAPTER 32
MULTIPLE ABNORMAL LABS CASE PRACTICE

THE PREVIOUS CHAPTERS discussed the approach to **isolated** lab abnormalities, which can be challenging in and of itself. Algorithms can guide the workup of isolated lab abnormalities. However, algorithms can lead you astray when there are **multiple** abnormal labs. Focusing on one lab at a time might miss a single underlying diagnosis causing all the abnormal test results.

Clinicians call these situations the **"Occam's Razor versus Hickam's Dictum"** challenge. Occam's razor attempts to explain all abnormalities with one underlying cause, whereas Hickam's Dictum states multiple etiologies can occur simultaneously. You'll need to consider both perspectives and reflect on which is more convincing in any given case.

Applying Occam's Razor can be particularly challenging for new clinicians. You'll need to develop pattern recognition skills to improve at this clinical reasoning exercise.

This chapter will share case vignettes with multiple lab abnormalities to develop your pattern recognition skills. Each of these can be answered with a single underlying condition. Since reference ranges aren't included here, I've put up and down arrows to show which direction the abnormality is. Test yourself further with the cases that famous internist Dr. Bob Centor presents on his YouTube channel, *Unremarkable Labs*.

PATTERN RECOGNITION PRACTICE WITH ABNORMAL LABS

What condition do you think is most likely causing the following lab derangements?

(1) Hgb 9.0↓, platelets 90k↓, AST 300s↑, ALT normal, total bilirubin 3↑ in a patient complaining of fatigue/lightheadedness. They deny a history of alcohol use or liver disease.

(2) Hgb 9.5↓, platelets 90k↓, AST 300s↑, ALT normal, total bilirubin 3↑ in an *ill-appearing sepsis patient* who is found to have *elevated PT/PTT*.

(3) Creatinine 2.5↑, AST 700s↑, ALT 100s, in a patient complaining of muscle aches.

(4) WBC 60K↑, Hgb 9.3↓, platelet 43↓ in a patient complaining of weight loss and bleeding gums.

(5) WBC 20K↑, AST/ALT 200s↑, TBili 6↑, Alk Phos 300s↑ in a patient complaining of RUQ pain and fevers.

(6) Na 128↓, K 4.0, CO2 12↓, AG 24↑, Glucose >500 in a diabetic patient complaining of nausea and vomiting.

(7) Na 128↓, K 5.6↑, and elevated eosinophils in a patient complaining of progressive fatigue and a BP of 90s/50s.

(8) Na 132↓, K 6.5↑, CO2 13↓, Creatinine 7.0↑, Ca 7.4↓ in a patient with previously diagnosed CKD stage III.

(9) AST/ALT 1000+, bilirubin 2↑, alk phos 120 in a recently immigrated patient with abdominal pain.

(10) Hgb 11.0↓, WBC 2.0k↓, Platelets 30k↓ in a patient with fever and petechiae.

(11) AST/ALT 2000s↑, INR 3.0↑, Ammonia 100 μmol/L↑ in a patient presenting with jaundice and confusion.

PATTERN RECOGNITION ANSWERS:

---

(1) Hgb 9.0↓, platelets 90k↓, AST 300s↑, ALT normal, total bilirubin 3↑ in patient with 1 week of fatigue? If this patient had these findings chronically or had a history of ETOH use, the most likely cause would be cirrhosis and impaired liver function. However, when these labs are noted acutely, the highest concern would be **a hemolytic anemia.** Think of a hemolytic anytime you see anemia *plus* elevated AST and bilirubin, which suggests RBCs are being broken down (hemolyzed).

When you also note **low platelets,** the concern is more focused on the **"MAHA/TMA" category of hemolyzing conditions** (TTP, DIC, HELLP, etc.). In MAHA (*microangiopathic* hemolytic anemia) disorders, there is some *external* process resulting in platelet clumping in small blood vessels (capillaries and arterioles). The "rough" vessels then shear the RBCs that pass through, destroying them (hemolysis) and forming **schistocytes** (torn-up RBCs). The result we see, and the pattern to look out for, is **anemia and thrombocytopenia + elevated bilirubin and AST.** Sometimes the lab will call you and say they can see schistocytes, which are pathognomic for MAHA/TMA. None of the MAHA conditions are benign, so refer these patients to the ED.

(2) Hgb 9.5↓, platelets 90k↓, AST 300s↑, ALT normal, total bilirubin 3↑ in a critically ill patient who is found to have elevated PT/PTT as well? **The answer is DIC.** This illustrates how another dangerous MAHA disorder (DIC) might present.

(3) Creatinine 2.5↑, AST 700s↑, ALT 100s in a patient complaining of muscle aches? **The answer is rhabdomyolysis.** Remember that AST is an intracellular enzyme seen in *many* cells throughout the body, not just liver cells but also RBCs (which is why hemolysis raises AST) and muscle cells in this case. Takeaway point: whenever you see AST much more elevated than ALT, consider alcohol use *as well as* some sort of *cell lysis* problem. Try to figure out which cell type or the location it is coming from (liver cell, red blood cell, muscle, heart, etc). Each cell

type in lysis will leave its own signature, like an elevated troponin in myocardial cell death.

(4) WBC 60K↑, Hgb 9.3↓, platelet 43↓ in a patient complaining of weight loss and bleeding gums? **Heme-Onc malignancy like leukemia.**

(5) WBC 20K↑, AST/ALT 200s↑, TBili 6↑, Alk Phos 300s↑ in a patient complaining of RUQ pain and fevers? This suggests a "cholestatic injury pattern." With fever and WBC, we must think of **ascending cholangitis.** Others on DDx include ETOH hepatitis and decompensated cirrhosis.

(6) Na 128↓, K 4.0, CO2 12↓, AG 24↑, Glucose >500? The answer is **DKA.** The criteria for DKA is in the name. Diabetes is reflected by elevated sugars. Ketosis is reflected by the elevated anion gap. Acidosis is suggested by low bicarbonate. Hyponatremia in this situation is referred to as "pseudo-hyponatremia of hyperglycemia" and doesn't need to be worked up or managed aside from fixing the hyperglycemia.

(7) Na 128↓, K 5.6↑, and elevated eosinophils in a patient complaining of progressive fatigue and has a BP 90s/50s? The pattern of low Na and high K should make you think of **adrenal insufficiency.** If they have "bronze tan skin," think of Addison's disease.

Cortisol suppresses the eosinophil count. The presence of an elevated absolute eosinophil count in a hypotensive patient should immediately suggest adrenal insufficiency.

(8) Na 132↓, K 6.5↑, CO2 13↓, Creatinine 7.0↑, Ca 7.4↓ patient? These findings suggest **ESRD** and the need for **emergent dialysis** (for hyperkalemia and acidosis). Common lab abnormalities seen in ESRD or those who missed dialysis are hyperkalemia, metabolic acidosis, and hypocalcemia.

(9) AST/ALT 1000+, bilirubin 2↑, alk phos 120 in a recently immigrated patient with abdominal pain? This is a **hepatocellular** pattern of injury and, in this case, suggests **acute hepatitis.**

(10) Hgb 11.0↓, WBC 2.0k↓, Platelets 30k↓ in a patient with fever and petechiae. This may suggest **aplastic anemia and bone marrow failure.** Fever in patients with neutropenia is high risk as these patients are considered immunocompromised.

(11) AST/ALT 2000s↑, INR 3.0↑, Ammonia 100 μmol/L↑ in a patient with jaundice and confusion. This may indicate **acute liver failure.**

———

In conclusion, when you have patients with multiple "red-colored abnormal test results," the best practice is to make a DDx. Brainstorm for conditions that could cause all the abnormalities seen. Then, consider what would be the most likely causes if multiple things were at play. Of all these possibilities, which seems most consistent with the patient's presentation?

CHAPTER 33
THE TEST IS NEGATIVE, NOW WHAT DO I DO?

MANY NEW GRADUATES hope their patient's test results return negative, thinking it will simplify decision-making. However, negative test results can give new clinicians a false sense of security. This is a classic pitfall seen in our M&M committee. Three "negative result" scenarios are prone to deceiving inexperienced clinicians.

First is the normal test result that is *deceptively* **normal**. There may be clinical contexts where you'd expect an *abnormal* result, and a normal test result is concerning. The patient with a "normal PTH" in the face of hypocalcemia has hypoPTH because you'd expect an *elevated* PTH. Consider also the normal hemoglobin and hematocrit (H/H) in the patient who reported having a large bloody bowel movement before arrival. The H/H drop can lag several hours before it reflects the true clinical picture.

The second type of situation involves radiology results for "clinical diagnosis conditions." New grads commonly fail to grasp the gravity of radiology reports that don't sound too concerning at first glance. Be especially careful when the radiologist comments, "clinical correlation required," as this conveys they are limited in how much they can help us make progress on the case. Here are a few classic examples:

- **A patient with low back pain, bilateral leg sciatica, and groin tingling** gets an MRI with this result: "Central disc herniation with effacement of the thecal nerve roots." Radiologists are taught **not** to explicitly write the diagnosis cauda equina syndrome because herniated discs are extremely common, of unknown chronicity, and impossible to say whether the compression against nerves is causing any symptoms. The clinician must see the whole clinical picture and realize that this is indeed cauda equina syndrome and needs emergent surgery.

- **A diabetic patient presents with pain, redness, and swelling in the right thigh**, with a CT result that notes, "Fat stranding, skin thickening, and subcutaneous emphysema. Query skin opening or drainage. Clinical correlation is required." Again, we must recognize that this is describing necrotizing fasciitis without saying the words directly.

- **A patient presents with neck pain after a car accident and has gone on to develop acute persistent vertigo.** A CT angiogram notes, "Small caliber of the right vertebral artery is intermittently identified over its expected course. This may be due to normal congenital variation of a dominant left vertebral system or may represent the sequelae of an age-indeterminate dissection." Whenever radiologists give us a DDx, the safest thing is to assume the worst: this is an acute dissection and since the patient has symptoms of cerebellar dysfunction, he may be suffering from a stroke, as was the case in this real closed malpractice claim.[1]

The last situation involves a negative test result but it **lacks the necessary sensitivity** to rule out the condition. These are also incredibly common sources of medical decision-making errors for new graduates. The practice cases next will illustrate these situations.

CASE PRACTICE: TEST NEGATIVE MISSES

I will provide the patient's presentation and the negative test result. Your job is to reflect on the DDx that remains, the limitations of the testing in assessing those possibilities, and what your next steps would be. Bonus points if you can identify the risks of missing the condition — in other words, why it matters for us not to miss these occult conditions. The answers will be listed below.

---

(1) A classic board question: 30-year-old male falls off a bike with a FOOSH injury (fall on outstretched hands), complaining of hand/wrist

---

1. https://expertwitness.substack.com/p/locked-in-syndrome-chiropractor-adjusts

pain. Hand + wrist X-rays are negative. What DDx remains possible, and how will you manage this patient? What are the risks of missing this Dx?

(2) 75-year-old female falls on her R hip, her hip X-rays are negative, but she cannot walk.

(3) 19-year-old autistic male presents with "RLQ abdominal pain," labs and CT abdomen pelvis are negative.

(4) 58-year-old female presents after a biking injury, landing on the L knee, she has pain, swelling and limited ROM, but X-rays are negative.

(5) 25-year-old female presents with acute LLQ abdominal/pelvic pain, intermittent waves for the past three hours, US read as simple 5cm L ovarian cyst with otherwise good flow to the ovary and no signs of bleeding.

(6) 19-year-old college student male presents over winter break with headache, malaise, and toxic-appearing. His roommate is sick with similar symptoms. Strep, flu, Covid-19 PCR, CBC, and BMP are all negative. (Sick contacts = must be viral, right? Not necessarily…)

(7) 58-year-old male falls from a ladder hitting his head, complaining of headache and nasal congestion since then. CT head is negative.

(8) 35-year-old female presents with acute onset severe headache and neck pain with onset last night, the symptoms have since resolved, and she comes requesting a work note. Non-contrast CT head is negative. (Resolving pain = reassuring feature? Not always…)

(9) 50-year-old male presents with chest pain, L arm pain, numbness tingling, and palpitations. EKG showing AFib, HR 80s, no ischemic changes, labs, and CXR is negative.

(10) 75-year-old male presents with neck pain and bilateral arm paresthesias since a rear impact MVC, CT head and neck without fracture, just showing arthritic changes to the neck.

(11) 35-year-old female presents with significant dyspnea, but her lungs are clear, and her CXR is negative.

Answers:

(1) A classic board question: 30-year-old male falls off a bike with a FOOSH injury: DDx still includes **occult scaphoid fracture**, with a risk of non-union, chronic pain, and disability if missed. If snuffbox tenderness is present, put the patient into a thumb spica splint and have them follow up with their PCP for a recheck. The PCP can consider repeating X-rays or advanced imaging if there is a high clinical concern.

(2) 75-year-old female falls on her R hip, her hip Xrays are negative, but she cannot walk: DDx still includes **occult hip fracture**, pelvis fracture, or back pathology (lumbar fracture/disc herniation/cauda equina syndrome). If there is clinical concern for hip fracture (significant pain, can't walk, can't range of motion hip well, pain with axial load or logrolling), the standard of care is to follow with a CT or MRI to evaluate further. Diagnosing a "hairline hip fracture" is important because an orthopedic surgeon can put a pin to fix it if caught early. If it is missed and the patient bears weight, causing the fracture to displace, it will require total hip replacement (and its associated increased morbidity/mortality). If the patient cannot walk, she will likely need admission even if advanced imaging is negative.

(3) 19-year-old autistic male presents with "RLQ abdominal pain," labs and CT abdomen pelvis are negative: DDx still includes missed appendicitis and testicular torsion. **Appendicitis** can be missed on CT if the patient presents soon after the symptoms start, and it can also be missed in thin patients because fat is necessary to see inflammatory stranding. **Testicular torsion** should be considered in any male patient with communication barriers (children, autism, etc.) presenting with "abdominal pain" or vomiting. I would perform a GU exam and check the cremaster reflex. If normal, I explain that appendicitis can be missed early in the course and they need a repeat exam within 12-24 hours if they have persistent pain.

(4) 58-year-old female presents after a biking injury, landing on the L knee, has pain, swelling and limited ROM. However, X-rays are negative: the DDx still includes **knee dislocation and spontaneous reduction (with vascular injury)**, **occult tibial plateau fracture** (requires CT scan), **patellar/quadriceps tendon rupture** (check for ability to perform knee extension), and of course the internal knee derangements like ligament/meniscus tears. Last, it is classically taught that **hip pathology** can manifest with knee pain and vice versa, so do a good hip exam.

(5) 25-year-old female presents with acute LLQ abdominal/pelvic pain, intermittent waves for the past three hours, US read as simple 5cm L ovarian cyst with otherwise good flow to the ovary and no signs of hemorrhage: DDx still includes **ovarian torsion**, **PID/TOA**, and **diverticulitis**. Ultrasound's sensitivity is much lower than expected for detecting decreased ovarian blood flow. Whenever you note an adnexal structure like an ovarian cyst to be reported as **over 4cm**, and the patient has significant pain in that region, consider consulting gynecology even if it is read as negative for torsion. Patients can have intermittent torsion that can be missed but still is time sensitive to be addressed. For further study, read the excellent summary article, "Dispelling 5 Ovarian Torsion Myths," by Dr. Brit Long.

(6) 19-year-old college student male presents over winter break for headache, malaise, and toxic-appearing. His roommate is sick with similar symptoms. The testing all results negative. Sick contacts = must be viral, right? DDx still includes **bacterial meningitis**, **sexually transmitted infections**, and **carbon monoxide poisoning**, which can cause nonspecific "viral sounding" symptoms and have positive sick contacts. Clinical evaluation with a thorough H&P is an excellent place to start when considering these entities.

(7) 58-year-old male falls from a ladder hitting his head, complaining of headache and rhinorrhea since then. CT head is negative: DDx still includes **occult basilar skull fracture**, which can be missed in half of CT scans if they are not significantly displaced. Consider this whenever you

hear of trauma resulting in a "runny nose" or "liquid coming from the ear." Perform a good exam for basilar skull fx signs (battle signs, raccoon eyes, hemotympanum, etc.). Take the reported "rhinorrhea or otorrhea" (which might be a CSF leak) and check it for fingerstick glucose, beta-trace protein, or a beta-2 transferrin test. Nasal congestion will test negative for these things, and CSF will test positive. If concerned, an easy first step is to call the radiologist to ask about re-formatting with thin slices reported to give 25% improved sensitivity.

(8) 35-year-old female presents with acute onset severe headache and neck pain the prior night, the symptoms have since resolved, and she comes requesting a work note. Non-contrast CT head is negative. Resolving pain = reassuring feature? DDx still includes a **cervical artery dissection** and a **subarachnoid hemorrhage (SAH)**. These are expected to improve with time, and CT scan will only reliably exclude a SAH if scanned within **6** hours of the start of symptoms. Suppose the story sounds like a subarachnoid hemorrhage and the patient presented in a delayed fashion. In that case, the CT scan is classically followed with a lumbar puncture (LP), though some experts are now recommending a CT angio approach instead of LP. This is an area of ongoing debate.

(9) 50-year-old male presents with chest pain, L arm pain, numbness, tingling, and palpitations. EKG shows AFib, HR 80s, no ischemic changes, labs, and CXR are negative: DDx still includes **aortic dissection and pulmonary embolism**, for which the patient would need a CT angio if there is clinical concern. **Pericardial effusion** can also be missed, as well as AFib plus limb pain suggesting the possibility of an **embolism with an ischemic limb**. Perform a thorough neurovascular exam whenever patients have extremity pain, numbness, or tingling.

(10) 75-year-old male presents with neck pain and bilateral arm paresthesias since a rear impact MVC, CT head and neck without fracture, just showing arthritic changes to the neck: The concern would be a **spinal cord syndrome** like central cord syndrome and would require an MRI. The trauma can be minor, and elderly patients with arthritis and hyper-extension injuries are at exceptionally high risk. A **neck artery dissection** could also cause these symptoms and be missed on a non-contrast scan.

• • •

(11) 35-year-old female presents with significant dyspnea, but her lungs are clear, and CXR is negative: DDx still includes common conditions like **pulmonary embolism, hemoglobinopathies** (anemia, CO poisoning, etc.), **acidosis** (e.g., DKA), **cardiovascular pathology** (CHF, pulmonary HTN, coronary ischemia/angina), and **neuromuscular weakness** (like myasthenia gravis), among many other conditions.

———

THE TAKE-AWAY LESSON

In short, don't let negative testing turn your brain off. You'll eventually find it helpful to **refine your approaches.** The Clinical Problem Solvers have shared schemas like *an approach to abdominal pain when imaging is negative.*[2] You will also find yourself developing more unique, situational differentials like these.

You can **protect yourself in your medical decision-making and charting** with a simple phrase like, "Testing for the patient came back unremarkable — I considered alternative and occult pathologies, but none seem likely based on the clinical picture and my exam at this time."

The last key pitfall regarding negative testing is **how you communicate the results with your patients**. The novice clinician might tell their patients, "Your tests came back negative, so there is nothing wrong with you." This will cause patients to ignore their symptoms if things worsen.

Our tests are imperfect. A better phrasing would be, "Your tests came back negative, so I can't say for certain what is causing your symptoms. We can still try treatment for my suspected diagnosis of XYZ. However, I want you to closely monitor your symptoms at home and go to the ED if anything worsens."

---

2. Geha, Rabih. "DX Schema – GI." The Clinical Problem Solvers, December 28, 2019. https://clinicalproblemsolving.com/reasoning-content/dx-schema-gi/.

CHAPTER 34

A CLINICAL APPROACH TO EKGS

I HAVE ALWAYS ASKED rotating students and new graduates, "What topics would you **most** want to have covered in a guidebook?" EKG interpretation is one of the most frequently requested topics. Many new graduates do not feel comfortable interpreting their EKGs in practice.

You have all heard about the importance of a systematic EKG approach and have likely been taught multiple methods. The method taught in textbooks and schools focuses on EKG analysis in a vacuum, but this is not how it is done in practice. In the real world, this is how we assess EKGs:

Step 1: Who is the patient — Age and sex? Chief complaint? Stable or unstable?

The first step in interpreting an EKG is not even involving the EKG. First and foremost, you need to know who the patient is, their vital signs, and their chief complaint. This background information colors everything in your EKG assessment. The same EKG will require a different evaluation if the patient is there for chest pain versus syncope.

Assuming the patient is stable, you can continue to the "traditional" EKG systematic interpretation below.

Step 2: **Systematic EKG Interpretation** — Identify all abnormalities.

(A) Rate — rhythm — axis — these basics will be reviewed shortly.

(B) Wave morphologies and intervals — are any of the waves or intervals too tall/short or too wide/narrow?

(C) Are there any **ischemic** findings or patterns present? Are any **other concerning patterns** present using a specific *search pattern* based on the chief complaint?

The above, "Step 2," is traditionally covered in school. If you don't have a good conceptual understanding of this section, skip ahead to "A Review of the Basics" in a couple of pages. If you understand these steps, continue to steps 3 through 5, which are typically not taught in grad school.

One point to emphasize: we use the above *systematic* approach to identify *all* abnormalities. Otherwise, you will be prone to stop prematurely after identifying your first abnormality.

You then reformulate these abnormalities into clinically relevant phrasing. For example, your initial impression might be, "I see something odd with the T waves," but you should then re-phrase it into the more precise "There are precordial T-wave inversions most localized to V1-V3").

Step 3: **Compare to prior EKGs:**

Are these findings new or old? This is a crucial step that many new graduates forget. Many patients have several abnormalities on their EKG that stress new grads until they realize it's simply their baseline.

Step 4: **What is the *most* prominent new finding that we have identified?**

Your systematic approach may have identified four abnormalities with the EKG, but which is the most striking? This will be the center of gravity you use to solve the case. We will cover this in the next chapter, but realize that this prominent finding (e.g., ST segment elevation) is *the starting point*, not a final diagnosis.

Step 5: Make progress from the main EKG finding to a diagnosis.

You need to take that prominent finding and generate a DDx to guide the next steps to determine the cause. Even things like ST segment elevation that most people automatically associate with a STEMI can frequently be caused by conditions like pericarditis, benign early repolarization, and several other conditions.

You can progress towards the final diagnosis by *analyzing the subtle EKG features* that might give you clues (e.g., are there reciprocal findings?). Often more important are the *next clinical evaluation steps* like history, exam, and testing needed to make sense of the EKG findings.

That is the overview of clinical EKG interpretation. Next, we will review the basics in further detail, and the following chapters will dissect the most important categories of EKG findings you'll need to know.

A REVIEW OF THE BASICS

The following are the basic steps of EKG interpretation that most grad schools cover well. I've included a review here for those who want a quick refresher.

RATE

There are several ways to determine the rate quickly. If it looks regular, I look at the rate printed on the top of the EKG and trust it if it matches the patient's vital signs. If it is irregular or doesn't feel right, you can use the commonly taught methods of counting the number of big boxes between two QRS complexes (300-150-100-75-60...) when the rate is fast, or counting the total number of QRS complexes and multiplying by six if the rate is slow.

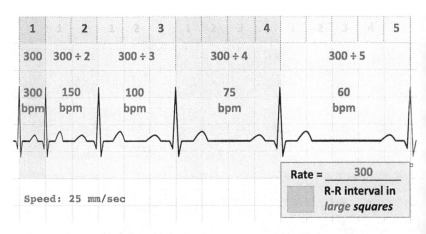

LITFL, Big box counting method, with permission.

RHYTHM

Does it look obviously to be normal sinus rhythm (NSR)? Great, you're done and can go to the next step.

If it's not NSR, scrutinize your rhythm strip (the single lead continuous strip on the bottom). Find every P wave and check if there is a QRS after each. Find every QRS complex and check for a P wave before each. While you're here, does the PR interval look normal and the same between each?

If you've identified an abnormal rhythm, you only have **three different**

184

possible sites of rhythm origin outside of the SA node. It's either an **atrial rhythm**, a **junctional rhythm**, or a **ventricular rhythm.**

(1) Atrial rhythms (AFib, Aflutter, PACs, MAT, etc.) most commonly have the signature of **variable, irregular, or absent P waves** and a **narrow complex QRS**. The QRS is narrow because these impulses originate above the AV node and go through the His-Purkinje Bundle. A common exception would be a bundle branch block, which can widen the QRS even in an atrial rhythm.

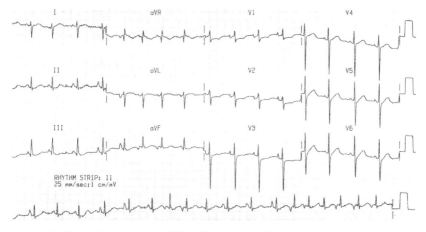

Multifocal atrial tachycardia, LITFL, with permission. Note the rhythm strip on the bottom with variable appearance of P waves and a narrow QRS.

(2) Junctional rhythms are the second potential site of electrical impulse origination. What is the "junction?" This refers to the **AV node** and the **His Purkinje bundle**. These structures can also generate electrical impulses that go down to the ventricles. However, they only do so when they aren't getting signals from the atria, as in severe bradycardia, SA node arrest, complete heart block, hyperkalemia, or medication toxicity (e.g., beta-blocker overdose). This is why they are called junctional "escape rhythms" and considered a safeguard for the heart. Whenever you see a *new onset* junctional rhythm, think of it as something serious impairing the SA node or conduction to the ventricles.

Since they use the His Purkinje bundle, junctional rhythms are also characterized by a **narrow QRS**. They tend to produce a heart rate between **40 and 60**. These rhythms will have **abnormal appearing P waves**, absent P waves, or no correlation between the P waves and QRS complex in the case of a heart block.[1] The P waves can also appear "retrograde" (flipped appearance because it has the opposite axis).

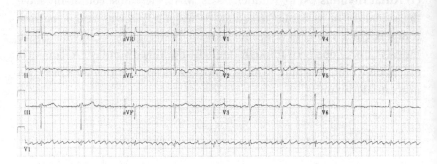

EKG with coarse AFib, complete heart block, and a junctional escape rhythm with a HR of 60. AFib plus a regular rhythm is characteristic of digoxin toxicity. LITFL.

(3) Ventricular rhythms (ventricular escape rhythm) are the last potential site of electrical impulse origination and the most concerning. They suggest a failure of the SA node and the AV node. They are seen with the same causes as junctional rhythms, like sinus arrest, complete heart blocks, and hyperkalemia. Consider a ventricular origin rhythm if you see a **wide QRS complex**, absent P waves, or a dissociation between P waves and the QRS (e.g., complete heart block). They tend to produce a heart rate between **20-40 bpm**, and **can deteriorate** into ventricular tachycardia or ventricular fibrillation.

---

1. https://litfl.com/junctional-escape-rhythm-ecg-library/

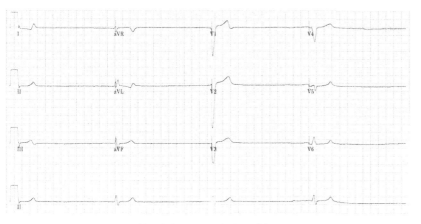

Ventricular escape rhythm, LITFL

Ventricular tachycardia and ventricular escape rhythms have distinct causes. Ventricular tachycardia (a fast and wide complex EKG) is very concerning as the most common cause is **myocardial ischemia / acute coronary occlusion**.

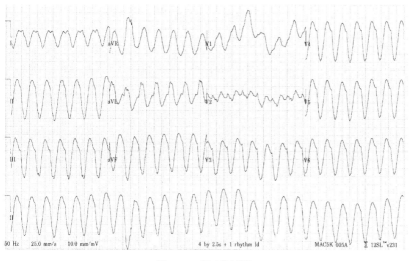

Monomorphic VT, LITFL

AXIS

What is the overall direction of energy as it makes its way through the heart? We compare and contrast each lead's positive/negative tracings to understand the overall energy direction. Leads I and aVF are frequently used because they are perpendicular to each other and in an X and Y axis.

Determining an abnormal axis can help us clinically. Consider a rightward deviated axis in a patient with dyspnea. This suggests the right side of the heart is under strain and requiring more energy, thus changing the vector of electrical impulse. The DDx for this would be pulmonary embolism if acute, and pulmonary hypertension (with a wide DDx) if chronic.

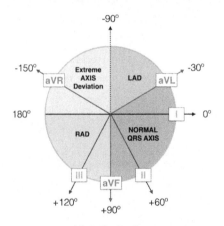

Life in the fast lane

Lead 1	Lead aVF	Quadrant	Axis
POSITIVE	POSITIVE		Normal Axis (0 to +90°)
POSITIVE	NEGATIVE		**Possible LAD (0 to -90°)
NEGATIVE	POSITIVE		RAD (+90° to 180°)
NEGATIVE	NEGATIVE		Extreme Axis (-90° to 180°)

Life in the fast lane

WAVE MORPHOLOGIES AND INTERVALS:

Does anything look too big or small, too wide or narrow?

This section is best explained with numerous pictures and examples outside this chapter's scope. Check out Life in the Fast Lane's website for a fantastic review.

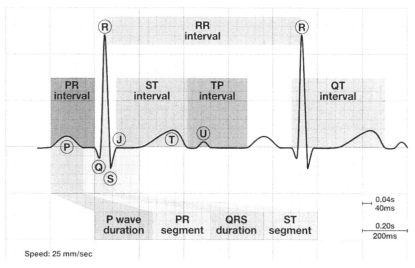

Life in the fast lane

ISCHEMIC PATTERNS

This generally would include your assessment for ST-segment elevation or depression, peaked or flipped T waves, pathologic Q waves, and poor R wave progression. Unique or atypical EKG patterns can suggest ischemia that wouldn't fit into the above classic changes, as summarized in the table below. If you note any of these, get help and transfer to the ED.

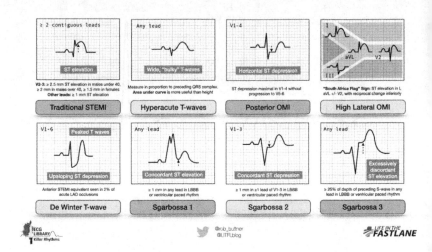

≥ 2 contiguous leads	Any lead	V1-4	I, aVL, V2, III
ST elevation	Wide, "bulky" T-waves	Horizontal ST depression	"South Africa Flag" Sign
V2-3: ≥ 2.5 mm ST elevation in males under 40, ≥ 2 mm in males over 40, ≥ 1.5 mm in females. Other leads: ≥ 1 mm ST elevation	Measure in proportion to preceding QRS complex. Area under curve is more useful than height.	ST depression maximal in V1-4 without progression to V5-6	"South Africa Flag" Sign: ST elevation in I, aVL +/- V2, with reciprocal change inferiorly
Traditional STEMI	**Hyperacute T-waves**	**Posterior OMI**	**High Lateral OMI**
V1-6 — Peaked T waves	Any lead	V1-3	Any lead — Excessively discordant ST elevation
Upsloping ST depression	Concordant ST elevation	Concordant ST depression	
Anterior STEMI equivalent seen in 2% of acute LAD occlusions	≥ 1 mm in any lead in LBBB or ventricular paced rhythm	≥ 1 mm in ≥1 lead of V1-3 in LBBB or ventricular paced rhythm	≥ 25% of depth of preceding S-wave in any lead in LBBB or ventricular paced rhythm
De Winter T-wave	**Sgarbossa 1**	**Sgarbossa 2**	**Sgarbossa 3**

ECG LIBRARY / Killer Rhythms   @rob_buttner @LITFLblog   LIFE IN THE FASTLANE

THE SEARCH PATTERN FOR EACH CHIEF COMPLAINT

While interpreting the EKG, you need a targeted review for specific patterns based on the chief complaint.

For patients with dyspnea, seek out the classic S1Q3T3 pattern that might support right heart strain and PE. For patients with chest pain, scrutinize every ST segment and T wave for subtle changes.

Some teach the EKG search pattern of **"WOBBLER"** for the patient who presents with **syncope**—WPW, obstructed AV pathway, bifascicular block, Brugada, LV hypertrophy (HOCM), epsilon wave, or a repolarization abnormality (long QT, short QT).

As you study the chief complaints, focus on the patterns of pathologies that might manifest on the EKG. These are also great to document in your note to show you are thoroughly reviewing the EKG for the highest-risk pathology.

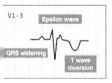

Arrhythmogenic Right Ventricular Dysplasia

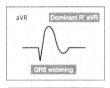

Sodium channel blockade

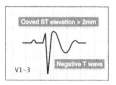

Brugada Syndrome

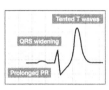

Hyperkalaemia

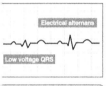

Massive pericardial effusion

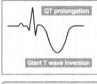

Intracranial haemorrhage

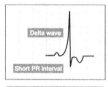

Wolff-Parkinson-White Syndrome

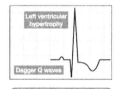

Hypertrophic Cardiomyopathy

CHAPTER 35
APPROACH TO "TOO FAST" AND "TOO SLOW" EKG BUCKETS

WHEN YOU GIVE an EKG to an experienced clinician, they will often speed through the steps of the last chapter in seconds and say something like, "Well, it looks like a narrow complex regular tachycardia, and I don't see any P waves... let's do XYZ." Even if they don't make a final diagnosis, they immediately hone in on the essence of the problem in a way that informs the next steps.

As you interpret EKGs, you should aim to determine the category if the diagnosis is not apparent. Luckily, there are only so many categories that exist:

TOO FAST

- Sinus tachycardia
- Narrow complex regular tachycardia
- Narrow complex irregular tachycardia
- Wide complex tachycardia

TOO SLOW

- Sinus bradycardia
- "Looks like a heart block of some kind"

NORMAL HEART RATE WITH PROMINENT FEATURE

- Wide QRS complex
- Long or short QT
- ST segment changes (elevated or depressed)
- T wave changes (peaked or inverted)
- New RBBB/LBBB

This chapter will review the key considerations that should come to mind once you have determined that a patient's EKG fits into one of the "too fast" or "too slow" buckets.

––––––

SINUS TACHYCARDIA (HR>100)

Whenever you identify sinus tachycardia, remember this: it's probably *not* a heart problem. There's usually something going on throughout the rest of the body that the heart is reacting to. There is a wide differential diagnosis, but the cause is usually apparent. We are not surprised by reactive tachycardia when patients present febrile, dehydrated, hypotensive, or after exercising.

But what if the cause is not clear based on the clinical picture? What is the DDx for more occult causes of sinus tachycardia that can manifest with nonspecific symptoms? This is the list to consider:

- **Hypovolemia** from occult **GI bleed or dehydration.**
- **Bacteremia** from things patients might not be forthcoming about, like **IVDU, endocarditis,** etc.
- **Pulmonary embolism.** This should always be on the DDx for unexplained tachycardia in a nonspecific presentation.
- These first three examples fall into the general category of "early shock states," in which there has been an insult to circulation but the blood pressure hasn't yet dropped because of the compensatory tachycardia. Let's review some other mechanisms for tachycardia next:
- **Endocrinopathy** like **hyperthyroidism,** or pheochromocytoma if episodic (pheo is incredibly rare, however).

- **Drug/alcohol intoxication or withdrawal**. These last categories are described by hyper-adrenergic or sympathetic surge states. Consider these more strongly if you note tachycardia *plus hypertension* (the opposite of what you'd expect in a shock state).
- **Primary cardiovascular causes** are possible, like myocarditis which classically causes unexplained and persistent tachycardia. An MI that impairs output would also result in sinus tachycardia. Usually, the clinical picture is informative here, and the patient doesn't just have an isolated sinus tachycardia.

The list goes much further, but the above will identify the most common causes of sinus tachycardia.

NARROW COMPLEX REGULAR TACHYCARDIA

A 35-year-old otherwise healthy man presents with acute onset palpitations without other complaints, vitals noting HR 165 and BP 130/80 with this EKG that you astutely note fits into the category of a narrow complex regular tachycardia without normal appearing P waves...[1]

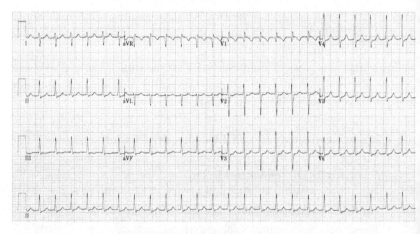

Life in the fast lane, SVT article, with permission

1. Buttner, Robert, Ed Burns. "Supraventricular Tachycardia (SVT)." *Life in the Fast Lane • LITFL* (blog), August 1, 2020. https://litfl.com/supraventricular-tachycardia-svt-ecg-library/.

This is a common clinical situation that you are likely to face. Like any other case, the first question is always, "**stable or unstable?**" If they are unstable, you will never go wrong with electricity (i.e., cardioversion, which is *synchronized* if they have a pulse).

The majority of these patients will be stable, and you are left with the following differential: **Paroxysmal SVT** (PSVT or AVNRT), **A-flutter** (especially if the HR is around 150), and **orthodromic WPW**. If you don't know these conditions well, ask for help before considering AV nodal blockers like adenosine and vagal maneuvers.

NARROW COMPLEX IRREGULAR TACHYCARDIA

A 65-year-old otherwise healthy female presents with gradual onset palpitations that she noted after several days of a productive cough, chills, and dyspnea. Vitals note a HR of 135 and BP of 102/68 with this EKG that you astutely note fits into the bucket of narrow complex *irregular* tachycardia without normal appearing P waves…[2]

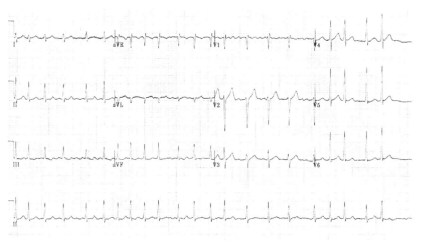

Life in the fast lane, AFib RVR

The vast majority of the time, this bucket will reflect atrial fibrillation with a rapid ventricular response (AFib with RVR). However, other

2. Buttner, Ed Burns and Robert. "Atrial Fibrillation." *Life in the Fast Lane* • LITFL (blog), August 1, 2018. https://litfl.com/atrial-fibrillation-ecg-library/.

alternatives could be multifocal atrial tachycardia in those with lung diseases like COPD, and atrial flutter with variable block (2:1, 3:1, etc.).[3]

AFib with RVR is incredibly common, but the average new graduate may not appreciate the numerous pitfalls in management. Here are some of the key concepts:

Concept 1 — Immediate management depends on whether the patient is **stable or unstable** (like always).

Concept 2 — General management considerations include **rate control vs. rhythm control** and **anticoagulation**. When considering rhythm control (converting AFib back to normal sinus rhythm), realize the risk of causing a stroke, especially if the patient has been in AFib for more than 48 hours. This is due to the risk of clot formation in the fibrillating atria that can dislodge once normal atrial contractions resume. For this reason, if there is any question about when the AFib started, many clinicians prefer to start with the safer rate control option. When considering rate control with agents like calcium channel blockers (CCBs) and beta blockers (BBs), you still must be mindful of whether these medications' negative effects on blood pressure (inotropy) and heart rate (chronotropy) might harm your patient. More on this below.

Stroke risk is estimated with the **CHA₂DS₂-VASc** score, and bleeding risk with the **HAS-BLED score** (or, physician gestalt). When necessitated by stroke risk, anticoagulation options depend on whether it's *valvular AFib* (warfarin preferred) or *non-valvular AFib* (DOACs are usually preferred if the patient can afford them).

Concept 3 — **Primary or secondary AFib**. You must always ask yourself whether this tachycardia is being driven simply by primary AFib or if there is some other *pathology* driving a *compensatory* tachycardia (akin to sinus tachycardia). Primary AFib responds well to rate control, whereas giving rate control to a patient in secondary AFib can be catastrophic.

Examples of secondary or compensatory AFib include patients who present with AFib with RVR *caused by* underlying sepsis, pulmonary emboli, hyperthyroidism, hypotension from GI bleed, or hypovolemia.

---

3. Julian, Hoevelmann, Viljoen Charle, and Chin Ashley. "Irregular, Narrow-Complex Tachycardia." *Cardiovascular Journal of Africa* 29, no. 3 (2018): 195–98.

In these situations, the best treatment for their AFib is to treat the underlying condition — by giving fluids and antibiotics to the septic patient or blood products to the GI bleeder. Imagine treating a septic patient with an IV beta blocker that quickly lowers their heart rate, removing the only thing that was keeping them from circulatory collapse.

How do you differentiate primary versus secondary AFib clinically? A lot of it is in the H&P and test results. If their only complaint is "palpitations since I stopped taking my metoprolol," (primary AFib) this is very different than the patient complaining of a productive cough, fevers, and dyspnea (secondary AFib).

Concept 4 — How will their heart handle rate-control agents? I have seen many patients with undiagnosed congestive heart failure and reduced ejection fraction (EF) decompensate after receiving calcium channel blockers for AFib with RVR. Always do a good physical exam for signs of heart failure, a chart check for their last echocardiogram, or a bedside echo if you have any concerns for CHF. If you have any concerns for a reduced EF, get help before starting treatment.

Concept 5 — The cardiologist's approach for long-term management considers options like ablation and much more. It seems the historical treatment of allowing patients to remain in atrial fibrillation chronically is going out of favor. Now, many experts recommend rhythm control to avoid harmful heart remodeling. Check out the Curbsider's podcast on atrial fibrillation for an excellent overview of the outpatient approach to management and when ablation comes into consideration.[4]

For a great hospitalist-based management of AFib, check out the PointOfCare website's summary.[5]

---

4. The Curbsiders. "#363 Afib: Rhythm Control, Catheter Ablation, Afib in the Hospital, and Left Atrial Appendage Closure," October 31, 2022. https://thecurbsiders.com/internal-medicine-podcast/363-afib-rhythm-control-catheter-ablation-afib-in-the-hospital-and-left-atrial-appendage-closure.
5. "Atrial Fibrillation - Inpatient Templates and Pearls." Accessed February 27, 2023. https://www.pointofcaremedicine.com/cardiology/afib.

WIDE COMPLEX TACHYCARDIA

A 65-year-old female with a history of CAD presents with chest pain, palpitations, and diaphoresis. Vitals note a HR of 160 and BP of 102/68 with this EKG that you astutely note fits into the category of a *wide complex regular tachycardia*...[6]

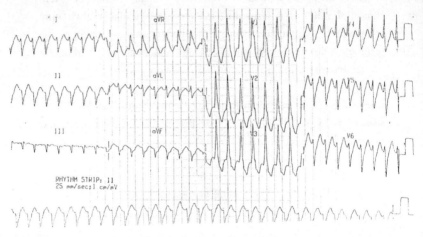

Life in the fast lane, with permission

Wide complex tachycardias are luckily not as common as narrow complex tachycardias. However, they are much higher risk and certainly warrant the involvement of your attending physician.

The differential diagnosis includes the following:

- **Ventricular tachycardia (V-tach)** — This is the most worrisome of these possibilities because it's often caused by coronary ischemia and results in instability.
- **Supraventricular rhythm with aberrancy** — For example, an SVT with a bundle branch block or WPW accessory pathway that slows down the depolarization of the ventricles causing the widened appearance of the QRS complex.

6. "Ventricular Tachycardia – Monomorphic VT • LITFL • ECG Library." Accessed February 27, 2023. https://litfl.com/ventricular-tachycardia-monomorphic-ecg-library/.

- **Toxic/metabolic** pathologies like hyperkalemia and sodium channel blockers can also cause these changes.

There are multiple systems to help distinguish the specific cause of a wide complex tachycardia, but they are not easy nor perfect methods.[7] The saying goes, "When in doubt, the safest thing to do is treat it as the most life-threatening possibility" (VTach). Get your attending or a cardiologist involved for help.

BRADYCARDIA (HR<60) KEY CONCEPTS

- **Concept 1** — Stable or unstable?
- **Concept 2** — Is it sinus bradycardia or a heart block of some sort? Review all of the P waves and QRS complexes as discussed.
- **Concept 3**—Most patients with sinus bradycardia will be stable. Our role is to determine whether there are any pathologic causes or if it is a benign condition.
- **Concept 4** — The DDx for common pathologic causes includes medications, ischemia, electrolytes (hyperK/hypoK), and more as noted below.
- **Concept 5** — "Benign" sinus bradycardia is suggested if the patient is otherwise young, healthy, athletic, lacks new symptoms like lightheadedness, and has an appropriate heart rate rise with ambulation. Elderly patients can also have benign bradycardia, but let chronicity and symptomatology guide you on when to be concerned.

Check out Dr. Foohey's fantastic bradycardia figure on the next page, summarizing it all.

---

7. Buttner, Robert, Ed Burns, and Robert Buttner and Ed Burns. "VT versus SVT." *Life in the Fast Lane* • *LITFL* (blog), January 1, 2021. https://litfl.com/vt-versus-svt-ecg-library/.

Approach to Bradycardia

1. First Steps

IV, O$_2$, Monitors, ECG
Pads on patient
Crash Cart in room
Unstable? Go to Step 2.

Unstable:
- HR generally <50
- Progressively worsening bradycardia
- Shock, SBP <90, Altered mental status
- SOB from CHF, Chest Pain

ECG:
- Bad block?
- Ischemia?
- HyperK?

2. Give Meds

Atropine 1mg IV q3-5min, max 3mg
Epinephrine 2-20mcg/min IV

Dopamine 5-20mcg/kg/min IV
Isuprel 2-10mcg/min IV

Set up Transcutaneous Pacing

1. Pads in AP position, connect ECG leads
2. Set pacemaker to **Demand** mode
3. Turn rate to 30bpm above intrinsic rate (start **60bpm**)
4. Set mA to **70mA** (estimate: 1mA/kg)
5. Start pacing: increase by 5mA every few seconds until pacing rate captured on monitor, then increase to 10% above this level (usually 5-10 mA above)
6. Confirm mechanical capture
7. Administer sedative & pain medication

Electrical Capture:

No Capture   Capture

Mechanical Capture:
- Feel femoral pulse
- HR on pulse oximeter
- Contractility on US

3. Consider DDx

Don't Let your Patients DIE: Drugs, Ischemia, Electrolytes

Drugs: ABCD
A: Amiodarone, Alpha Blocker
B: Beta Blockers
C: Calcium Channel Blockers
D: Digoxin
Organophosphates
Opioids
Sodium channel blockers

Ischemia
MI

Electrolytes
HyperK
HyperMg
HyperCa

Other
Myocarditis
Cardiomyopathy
Infiltrative disorders
↑ICP
Neurogenic Shock
Hypothyroid

Hypothermia
Anorexia
OSA
BRASH Syndrome
Lyme Disease
Syphilis

CHAPTER 36
APPROACH TO OTHER EKG BUCKETS

So far, we've delved into assessing patients with heart rates that are too fast or too slow. But what happens when the heart rate is normal? We can't let our guard down. There are a few other vital EKG buckets that warrant your attention.

In this chapter, we will focus on understanding and working up these high-risk findings:

- Wide-complex QRS
- Inverted T waves
- Long QT interval

WIDE QRS COMPLEX (AND A SLOW OR NORMAL HR)

A 75-year-old female with no known PMH presents with dyspnea, malaise, and generalized weakness. Vital signs note a BP of 170/105, a HR of 50, and you notice a wide-appearing complex on the cardiac monitor prompting an order that shows the following EKG.[1]

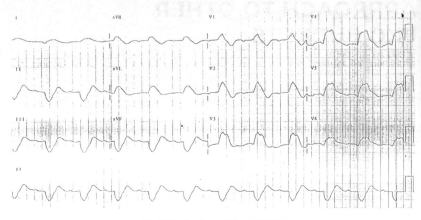

Life in the fast lane, with permission

You astutely note a wide complex EKG, but this time it is not a "wide complex *tachycardia*." Whenever you see a wide complex EKG with a normal or slow heart rate, this pattern should trigger consideration of **hyperkalemia** first and foremost, as it is an immediately life-threatening finding. Other possibilities include the following:

- **Ventricular escape rhythm** or **heart block.**
- Supraventricular rhythm with **aberrancy** (bundle branch block, WPW, etc.).
- **Sodium channel blockade** (e.g., TCA ingestion in a suicide attempt).
- **Metabolic/electrolyte** derangement.

INVERTED T WAVES

A 35-year-old female with no known PMH presents with chest pain and

1. Buttner, Robert, Ed Burns, and Robert Buttner and Ed Burns. "Hyperkalaemia." *Life in the Fast Lane • LITFL* (blog), August 1, 2018. https://litfl.com/hyperkalaemia-ecg-library/.

dyspnea. Vital signs note a BP of 98/64, a HR of 120, and you note the following EKG.[2]

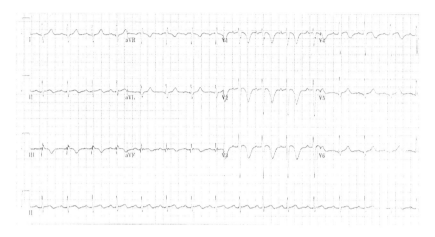

You immediately recognize the prominent T-wave inversions, which are mostly in the precordial leads and to a lesser extent in the inferior leads. Your search pattern also discovers the S1Q3T3 pattern, which suggests R heart strain. This clinical picture is highly suggestive of pulmonary embolism.

T-wave inversions should prompt consideration of a rather broad DDx:

- **Pulmonary embolism**, or any other cause of **right heart strain** (e.g., pulmonary hypertension) when the T wave inversions are noted over the R side of the heart (V1-V3).
- **Coronary ischemia** (e.g., "Wellen's pattern").
- **Intracranial events** like hemorrhage, raised intracranial pressure, etc.
- **Myocarditis**.
- **Takotsubo's cardiomyopathy**.
- **Juvenile** T-wave inversions.
- **HOCM**.
- **ARVC**.

2. Burns, Ed, Robert Buttner, and Ed Burns and Robert Buttner. "ECG Changes in Pulmonary Embolism." *Life in the Fast Lane • LITFL* (blog), August 1, 2020. https://litfl.com/ecg-changes-in-pulmonary-embolism/.

Many of these conditions can be sorted out with a good history and physical exam. If you have concerns about a specific cause, you further evaluate with testing as indicated.

LONG QT

A 53-year-old female with a history of depression and cannabinoid hyperemesis syndrome presents with intractable nausea and vomiting for several days and now feels extremely weak. The triage team pushes 8mg of IV ondansetron, and you note the following EKG while the patient faints in front of you.[3]

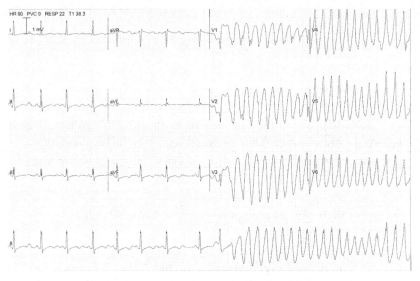

Life in the fast lane, with permission

What happened here? In the first half of the EKG, you should notice a particularly long QT. The DDx for long QT is listed below, but one that should immediately come to mind is electrolyte disturbances like **hypokalemia** and **hypomagnesemia** (commonly seen in vomiting). She was also on other home **medications that prolong the QT**. Since this patient was given a QT-prolonging nausea medication, she went into the unstable rhythm *Torsades de Pointes*. When Torsades is recognized in an unstable patient, the patient should be cardioverted (if pulses are present)

3. Buttner, Robert, Ed Burns, and Robert Buttner and Ed Burns. "Hypokalaemia." *Life in the Fast Lane* • *LITFL* (blog), April 24, 2021. https://litfl.com/hypokalaemia-ecg-library/.

or defibrillated (if pulseless) and given IV magnesium as soon as possible. Long QT is common enough that we will dive a bit deeper.

A **prolonged QT interval** can be appreciated even without checking the exact measurement by using the rule of thumb of where the T wave ends compared to the two surrounding QRS complexes ("RR interval"). If the T wave ends past the halfway point between the RR interval, it is a prolonged QT. In the above case, the T wave end almost overlaps the P waves, clearly a significant derangement. The reference ranges for the upper limit of normal are a QTc of 440ms for men and 460ms for women, with a **QTc >500 conferring the highest risk.**[4]

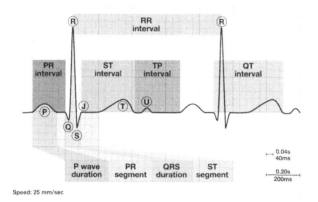

Source: Life In The Fast Lane Blog.

A few things should immediately come to mind whenever you notice a long QT. **First step: do no harm.** Do not make the QT even longer by using a QT-prolonging medication. Ondansetron is technically one of them, but very low risk when given at the usual dose of 4mg orally. Some of the other major classes of QT-prolonging medications include **anti-arrhythmics** (amiodarone, procainamide), **antibiotics** (macrolides, fluoroquinolones), **anti-psychotics** (haloperidol), **anti-depressants** (SSRIs),

---

4. Burns, Ed. "QT Interval." *Life in the Fast Lane* • LITFL (blog), August 1, 2020. https://litfl.com/qt-interval-ecg-library/.

anti-fungals (azoles), **opioids** (methadone), and importantly, many of the **anti-emetics.**[5]

For our patient case above, you can opt for nausea medications that won't prolong the QT, as detailed in the following diagram.

antiemetic pharmacology

Receptor being blocked:	D2 dopamine	M1 AcH	H1	5HT3 serotonin	QT	Sedation	Dose
Side-effects related to blocking this receptor	Extrapyramid. (e.g., akathisia, dystonia).	Sedation, delirium, dry mouth, urinary retention.	Sedation.	Few side effects.			
5-HT3 inhibitor							
Ondansetron				++++		None	8 mg IV *slowly*
Palonosetron				++++	None	None	0.25 mg IV
Esp useful in: Postoperative, chemo-induced. Often trialed as initial agent due to benign side-effect profile (primarily QT prolongation).							
Butyrophenones							
Droperidol*	++++		+				0.625 - 2.5 mg IV*
Haloperidol*	++++		+				1 - 5 mg IV/IM*
Esp useful in: Cannabinoid hyperemesis, postoperative, gastroparesis. QT only minimally elevated by low, antiemetic doses of these agents.							
Phenothiazines							
Prochlorperazine	++++	++	++				10 mg IV
Chlorpromazine	++++	++	++++	+			25 mg IV/IM
Promethazine	++	+++	++++				12.5-25 mg PO/IM
Prochlorperazine: especially useful for migraine.							
Olanzapine	+	+	+	++	None		2.5 mg IV/IM may repeat PRN
Broad-spectrum agent that is effectively a *combination* of ondansetron plus prochlorperazine. May be given PO, sublingually ODT, IM, or IV (FDA approved for IM administration but safe for slow IV push, similar to haloperidol). Data: impressive efficacy esp in chemo; good safety profile (no QT prolongation; low risk of extrapyramidal sx; sedation is main issue).							
Metoclopromide	+++			++		None	10-20 mg
Niche agent for: Gastroparesis, perhaps migraine. Not a great antiemetic. 10 mg is often *ineffective* for nausea/vomiting. Higher doses work better, but more extrapyramidal side-effects.							
Diphenhydramine		++	++++				25-50 mg
Dimenhydrinate					None		
Hydroxyzine							
Meclizine					None		
Niche agent for: Vestibular etiologies, Parkinsons disease.							

Internet Book of Critical Care emcrit.org/ibcc/antiemetic

Source: EMcrit.org IBCC Anti-emetic chapter, Dr Josh Farkas, with permission.

Second step: Ask yourself, why is the QT long? Many are medication or electrolyte-related. The rule of thumb is a **decrease** in the "heart's electrolytes" predisposes to it. Remember, vomiting classically causes a *hypo*kalemic hypochloremic metabolic alkalosis, and diarrhea can cause *hypo*magnesemia.

Here is the whole list of common causes of a long QT:

---

5. Berul, Charles. "Acquired Long QT Syndrome: Definitions, Pathophysiology, and Causes - UpToDate." Accessed December 31, 2022. https://www.uptodate.com.

- *Hypo*kalemia
- *Hypo*magnesemia
- *Hypo*calcemia
- *Hypo*thermia
- QT-prolonging medications or drugs (as noted above)
- Congenital long QT
- Increased intracranial pressure
- Myocardial ischemia

Third step: Correct the cause. Replete electrolytes and stop QT-prolonging medications and then repeat the EKG to confirm it has normalized.

––––––

USEFUL RESOURCES FOR DEEPER DIVES ON EKG INTERPRETATION

Where should you go to learn these basics and work through the different EKG topics? If you have a subscription to *EM:RAP* (Emergency Medicine Reviews and Perspectives), I've found their EKG content incredible. If not, try these fantastic resources freely available online:

- **Lifeinthefastlane.com:** The quintessential repository for all things EKG.
- **Dr. Smith's ECG blog** at http://hqmeded-ecg.blogspot.com: The expert on subtle ischemia patterns and case examples.
- Any lecture you can find online by ER **Dr. Amal Mattu,** a fantastic speaker whose specialty is cardiology in the ED.
- Any lecture you can find by cardiologist **Dr. Laurel Brown,** another wonderful speaker with Louisville lectures.

After you have learned the approaches to each EKG bucket, it's time for *practice, practice, practice.* Dr. Mattu has written fantastic books entitled *ECGs for the Emergency Physician I and II.* Practice with these challenge cases to solidify the concepts from this chapter.

––––––

With our sections on workup and interpreting test results complete, we will next turn our focus to safe prescribing practices.

CHAPTER 37
ACTION ITEMS

THE FOLLOWING action items can help you to order the right tests and interpret their results correctly:

- Use quick references to place the "**standard order sets**" for your patient's chief complaint.
- Use your **DDx and problem list** to remember other orders.
- Call a **radiologist** if you have a question on the best imaging study to order.
- Err toward ordering **more tests** in your first year.
- If your tests all come back negative, **pause** to consider if anything on your DDx might be missed because of tests with poor sensitivity. Document why you don't think those are present.
- For isolated lab abnormalities, **algorithms** are helpful for new graduates. Check out the algorithms on the Clinical Problem Solvers and other platforms.
- For patients with multiple lab abnormalities, consider if a **single condition** could be underlying them before working up each independently.
- Don't forget the **most dangerous results on the CBC**: Elevated WBC (think infection first), neutrophils under 500 (think immunocompromised), acute drop in hemoglobin, and platelets under 50k.
- Don't miss the **most dangerous results on the CMP:** Na under

120, K under 3 or over 6, Bicarb under 16, bilirubin over 3, calcium under 7 or over 14.

- Whenever you see **low bicarbonate**, there's a 99% chance of it being a **metabolic acidosis**. Look to the **anion gap** to characterize it as a HAGMA or a NAGMA. Then, work through the DDx to see which condition fits your patient's presentation. Treat the underlying condition.
- Whenever you see **high bicarbonate**, you'll need a **dedicated VBG** to see if it's a metabolic alkalosis or a respiratory acidosis with compensation.
- When you order an EKG, try to reach a **final diagnosis** or at least **categorize it into an "EKG bucket"** that will inform the DDx and the next steps in management.

Here are some **high-yield questions** to ask co-workers related to this section:

- What are the most commonly ordered diagnostic tests of our specialty?
- Which test results do you find the most challenging to interpret?
- How did you get comfortable interpreting them when you first started?
- What are the most common areas of confusion / mistakes you see from new grads working up patients?

PART SEVEN

HOW TO PRESCRIBE MEDICATIONS SAFELY

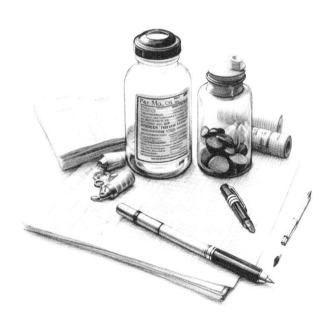

PRESCRIBING WOES

I always laugh when I recall a scene from the TV series *Scrubs*, where the intern JD asks Dr. Cox how to order acetaminophen and the safe dose. Dr. Cox responds, "You open their mouth, take a handful of it, and throw it at them. Whatever sticks is the right dose, Bambi."

The *Scrubs* writers perfectly captured the anxious feeling that new graduates get when faced with countless medications, dosing guidelines, interactions, and more. I felt the same and constantly second-guessed myself. One challenge with pharmacology is the incredible breadth and depth of knowledge available. Where should you begin?

Take some time to do the following preparatory actions to set yourself up for success:

1. **Make a medication shortlist:** Find your specialty's top twenty most prescribed medications. Google search, ChatGPT, or ask your new coworkers to generate the list. Review just the most clinically relevant details (i.e., risks, contraindications, dangerous side effects, and monitoring requirements). Consider creating your own quick-reference sheet, building off of the ones made by others online or in textbooks. I'll share an example table on the next page.
2. **Study the "safe prescribing habits":** We will review these practice essentials next chapter.
3. **Have a plan to answer the most common prescribing questions:** After a few weeks of practice, you'll notice the pattern of questions. "Are medications truly indicated for my patient? If so, what's the first-line agent? Is this first-line agent safe for my patient, or when should I consider second-line agents?" We will review the best ways to answer these questions and more.
4. **Get your pharmacist's number on speed dial:** Pharmacists are invaluable resources and have saved countless lives. Use them to their full potential!
5. **Download the best medication references to your phone:** UpToDate, Epocrates, and FirstLine (Antibiotic guidance based on local antibiograms, when available).

The following chapters will review the fundamentals. Before long, you'll be picking up on nuanced medication issues like this new graduate:

———

"I helped a patient when two other providers missed it. The patient came in reporting a chronic cough. She has been diagnosed with everything from bronchitis to GERD. She gave me a list of over five cough medications and antibiotics without improvement.

I reviewed her medication list and asked, 'How long have you been taking lisinopril?' She responded, 'About five months.'

'How long have you had this cough?'

'Five months…'

We stopped the lisinopril, and she called back later, saying the cough finally resolved. She was thrilled. I love this part of my job!"

NEW GRAD NP, FAMILY MEDICINE

TABLE 3.1 Chart of Hypertension Medications

Class of Drugs	Names, Dosing and Administration	Mechanism of Action / Indications	Adverse Effects/Toxicity	Warnings and Contraindications
Thiazide Type Diuretics	Chlorthalidone 12.5–25 mg/day Hydrochlorothiazide 12.5–25 mg/day Indapamide: 1.25 mg/day of indapamide	Inhibit sodium transport in the distal convoluted tubule cells of nephrons and decrease Na+ reabsorption, may have some vasodilating effects	Hypokalemia, hyponatremia, hyperuricemia, hyperglycemia, hyperlipidemia, hypomagnesemia occasionally, hypercalcemia sexual dysfunction in men	Potentially sulfonamide allergies Anuria
Loop Diuretics (used for heart failure and edema NOT first line for HTN) These are included in this chart and in the heart failure chart	Furosemide: oral dosage IV 20–40 mg once then titrate as needed max daily dose 600 mg/day Bumetanide (IV, po forms): initially Initial: 0.5–1 mg once daily and titrate (weight, fluid status) Torsemide Initial: 10–20 mg once daily; may increase gradually by doubling dose max is 200 mg/day Ethacrynic acid: oral dose: 50–200 mg/day in 1–2 divided doses, IV 50 mg or 0.5–1 mg/kg/dose	Inhibit Na-K-2 Cl carrier in ascending limb of loop of Henle, significantly reducing Na+ reabsorption	Profound diuresis with water and electrolyte depletion	Anuria Warning but not contraindication Sulfonamide ("sulfa") allergy unclear if cross-reactivity with nonantibiotic and antibiotic sulfonamides
Potassium sparing diuretics • Aldosterone antagonists • Amiloride and triamterene directly block sodium channels in principal cells of collecting ducts	Aldosterone antagonists Not first line for initial management • Eplerenone: Initial: 50 mg once daily can increase to 50 mg BID • Spironolactone: Initial: 25 mg once daily; titrate as needed based on response and tolerability up to 100 mg once daily Amiloride 5–10 mg in 1–2 divided doses (better tolerated than triamterene) Triamterene 100 mg po twice daily	Eplerenone Spironolactone inhibit the mineralocorticoid receptors in collecting ducts, which reduce urinary excretion of K+ and increases and Na and water reabsorption Amiloride and triamterene directly block sodium channels in principal cells of collecting ducts, which reduces K+ excretion into urine	All can cause hyperkalemia Spironolactone: gynecomastia, menstrual abnormalities, impotence, and decreased libido Triamterene can cause nephrotoxicity and increase kidney stone formation	Hyperkalemia Anuria Severe liver or kidney disease Caution with other drugs, which increase potassium including potassium supplements Caution with eplerenone and Addison disease

Example medication reference with high-yield bullet points. This figure comes from *Mind Maps in Medical Pharmacology,* by Jennifer Hofmann, DMSc., MS, PA-C, with permission.

CHAPTER 38
HABITS FOR SAFE PRESCRIBING

Most medication errors occur because of our fast-paced work environment. We are pushed to see an ever-increasing number of patients, and taking shortcuts can seem like a requirement. We skip things like reviewing the patient's entire medication list. We try to rely on memory for the correct dosage.

Shortcuts like these open everyone up to errors, but the risk is amplified for new graduates. If you can ingrain a few healthy "prescribing habits" from the beginning, you'll have an excellent defense against 95% of medication errors.

———

HABIT 1: "I will always strive for **a definitive diagnosis.**"

This may seem obvious, but everything hinges on this branch point. Prescribing medications is a serious intervention, and you should be as sure as you reasonably can that the patient needs them. Double-check they meet the criteria for diagnosis and medication management.

In patients without a confirmed diagnosis, prescribing nothing at all may very well be the best choice. As the famous Voltaire once said, "The art of medicine consists of amusing the patient while the body heals itself."

———

HABIT 2: "Every time I make **an unfamiliar diagnosis**, I'll look up the first-line treatment on a reliable reference."

For example, if you diagnose pelvic inflammatory disease, use a reference like **UpToDate** or **Epocrates** to search the **diagnosis keyword** to verify the first-line therapy, dosage, and duration.

When I say "unfamiliar," I am referring to *most* diagnoses you'll make in your first few months of practice. Once you've done this search enough times that it's burned in your memory, you can consider the diagnosis "familiar" enough not to double-check the first-line treatment details anymore. Habit 4 will also be a safeguard for this step.

––––––

HABIT 3: "Every time I consider prescribing **an unfamiliar medication**, I'll use a reference to review the contraindications, black box warnings, and required monitoring."

The reference suggests current PID treatment includes ceftriaxone, doxycycline, and metronidazole. Of these, you can't quite remember the details for doxycycline. You then dedicate an UpToDate or Epocrates search for the **dedicated medication page** to learn it should be avoided in pregnancy, prompting a pregnancy test (if you had previously forgotten to order one).

This is a frequently missed step by new grads. As someone new to the field, *most* medications you prescribe should be considered unfamiliar. UpToDate should be pinned to your home screen and left open most hours of the day!

––––––

HABIT 4: "When I finish researching, I'll **save the medication order** in my EMR with a descriptive **display name**."

New grads who rely on rote memory for future prescriptions are more prone to medication errors. Savvy clinicians can leverage the power of the EMR to help them overcome these types of mistakes.

While you have the medication order pulled up in your EMR (but *before* you hit enter/prescribe), **favorite the order** and **include the following descriptors**: the diagnosis, medication, and year you added the order favorite. For diagnoses that require multiple medications, include the relative number, like med 1 of 3. You can add a quick note like, "Check pregnancy test first," as well if you'd like. In the screenshot below, I've changed the display name in the highlighted section to, "PID Tx 1 of 3, Doxy x14 days, 2023"

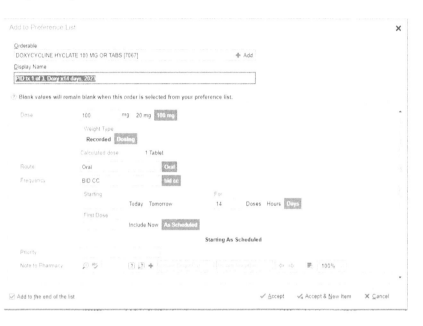

In future PID patients, simply typing "PID" into your medication order search will bring up all your saved PID medications with the verified dosing.

Including the year in the description helps keep your prescribing practices current. If it's been multiple years since you last looked up the saved order, search your reference again to see if the guidelines have changed, then update the year.

———

HABIT 5: "Before prescribing anything, I'll double-check **my patient's background medical information** — their PMHx, med list, and allergies — to ensure the medication is safe for them. **I'll also ensure their EMR med list is updated.**"

Your search above may have found the first-line treatment for a given diagnosis. Whether this medication is safe for the patient in front of you is an entirely different question. For example, pregnant patients or those with chronic organ dysfunction can't take many medications and need second or third-line therapies. An upcoming chapter will review the patient populations that pose the biggest challenge for prescribers.

The **drug interaction detector in EMRs is a lifesaver** because no human can memorize the thousands of potential interactions. However, it's only as good as the input it receives. Some clinicians skip this step, but you shouldn't make this mistake. Updating the EMR med list is an essential habit for safe prescribing.

HABIT 6: "Whenever I consider prescribing a **high-risk medication**, I'll first assess alternatives, use shared decision-making, and document my rationale."

Some medications are considered high-risk regardless of the patient population because of the possibility of severe or long-term adverse effects. New grads often don't have the experience to know which medications are high-risk. The next chapter will review these types of medications.

HABIT 7: "Whenever I feel **unsure** or in a **high-risk situation**, I'll get help by asking my attending physician or pharmacist."

For new grads unsure when it's appropriate to ask their attendings or pharmacists for help, this is a great time to do so. You should articulate why you need their help and the steps you've taken to develop a preliminary plan.

HABIT 8: "I'll **double-check each section** of the Rx before I hit sign."

The EMR often auto-populates every section of a prescription, and mistakes are easy to make if you don't double-check each section before you hit sign. For example, my EMR often defaults to #dispense 90 tabs, hidden at the bottom of the screen, even for some controlled substances.

———

In summary, integrate the following habits to become a safe prescribing pro:

1. Always strive for **a definitive diagnosis.**
2. Whenever you make **an unfamiliar diagnosis**, look up the **disease page** for the first-line treatment on a reliable reference.
3. For every **unfamiliar medication**, use a reference to double-check the clinically relevant details on the **dedicated medication page**.
4. **Save your medication orders** in your EMR with a descriptive 'display name' to let the computer remember these details for you.
5. **Know your patient** — Double-check their background medical information and **update the EMR med list** to ensure the interaction checker works.
6. Before prescribing a **high-risk medication,** first assess alternatives, use shared decision-making, and document your rationale.
7. **Get help** in high-risk situations or when unsure. Pharmacists are fantastic resources.
8. **Double-check each section** of the Rx before you hit sign.

CHAPTER 39
HIGHER-RISK
MEDICATION LIST

I REMEMBER ALL TOO WELL how overwhelming pharmacology was in PA school. We were exposed to hundreds of new medications, each with a textbook chapter describing countless drug details. For new graduates, it is easy to get lost in the details and fail to see the big picture: What medications are generally considered *safe* for most patients, and which have greater potential to cause *harm*?

I looked but didn't find a list like this in school or the few years after graduation. I have since learned of the *Institute for Safe Medication Practices,* which publishes a list of "High-Alert Medications in Acute and Ambulatory Care Settings."[1]

In this chapter, I'll do my best to summarize my list of higher-risk medications. Due to various experiences, my list has grown beyond the Institute's. Over the years, I've had numerous instructive calls from pharmacists saying, "Hey, that med is probably a poor choice, and here's why." I've also noticed a pattern of certain medications being culprits in bad outcomes in our morbidity and mortality committee.

I'd encourage you to pause and think critically before ordering the following medications. Double-check that they are truly indicated for the patient's diagnosis with a reliable reference, and look up whether alternatives exist. Many of these are indeed first-line and must be prescribed, and that's okay. The take-home message is that you must

---

1. Institute For Safe Medication Practices. "High-Alert Medications in Acute Care Settings," November 16, 2017. https://www.ismp.org/recommendations/high-alert-medications-acute-list.

understand **why** they are higher-risk medications so you can inform the patient and explain the reasons to stop taking the medication.

You might see some of these medications and think, "I'll never prescribe that drug; this is an irrelevant list to me." Even if a medication like cyclophosphamide might only be prescribed by an oncologist, you will still undoubtedly manage patients who have cancer and medications like these buried in their medical records. We need to recognize high-risk subspecialty meds and know their risks as well. If a patient presents with concerning symptoms, we need to know whether or not we should include adverse drug effects on the DDx.

––––––

HIGH-RISK MEDICATIONS IN GENERAL MEDICAL SPECIALTIES

TRAMADOL

Opiates, in general, are higher-risk medications, though we will review them in detail in two chapters. Tramadol is in its own unique category within the world of opiates. I trained in a center with toxicologists whose complaints about tramadol are nicely summarized in the articles "Tramadol, more like tramadon't" and "Don't prescribe tramadol."[2,3] So, what are the issues with tramadol?

First, the **efficacy** is **worse for treating pain** than alternatives, and even that weak efficacy is **inconsistent from patient to patient**. This is related to the mechanism of action. Tramadol inhibits serotonin and norepinephrine reuptake like SNRIs (e.g., Venlafaxine). It is tramadol's *metabolite* that has opioid effects. However, the conversion from tramadol to its opioid metabolite depends on the individual liver's cytochrome P450 enzymes (CYP2D6), and **this enzyme is widely variable from person to person**. Somewhere between 3-10% of Caucasians are poor metabolizers, resulting in minimal opioid effect, whereas others can be ultra-rapid metabolizers having a potent opioid effect. As a prescriber, you are gambling and don't know the impact on your patient. This is the same issue with **Codeine** and why many recommend against prescribing that as well.

As a whole, when compared to other analgesic medications, tramadol

2. Calello MD, Diane. "Tox & Hound: Tramadont." Accessed December 29, 2022. https://toxandhound.com/toxhound/tramadont/.
3. Morgenstern, Justin. "Don't Prescribe Tramadol." First10EM, May 13, 2019. https://first10em.com/tramadol/.

was found to be equally effective as acetaminophen for abdominal pain, worse than NSAIDs for biliary colic, and inferior to 5mg of hydrocodone and acetaminophen for relieving acute musculoskeletal pain.[4,5,6]

Because of the nonspecific effect on multiple receptors, tramadol can increase the risk of **serotonin syndrome**, respiratory depression, hypoglycemia, and hyponatremia. It also **lowers the seizure threshold** and should be avoided in patients with epilepsy or alcoholism.

One large propensity-matched observational cohort study in patients treated for osteoarthritis demonstrated an **association between tramadol use and increased all-cause mortality** compared to alternative agents.[7]

FLOUROQUINOLONES (E.G., CIPROFLOXACIN)

Quinolones present numerous risks, including musculoskeletal toxicity that can lead to tendonitis and **tendon rupture**, side effects on the central nervous system (e.g., headaches, confusion, seizures), **QT prolongation**, and a greater risk of **C. Diff** infection. They also have the potential to impact **connective tissues** in the body and contribute to aortic aneurysms, dissections, and retinal detachments. They have many **drug interactions**, and patients taking **calcium-containing liquids** simultaneously can render the quinolone ineffective.

Despite these issues, there are instances where no safe alternatives exist. In these situations, the risk of non-treatment must be weighed against the dangers of quinolone use. The **highest risk group** for issues like tendon rupture includes age >60, renal failure, diabetes, non-obese patients, and those using oral glucocorticoids. Counsel your patients on the risks, signs, and symptoms to look for adverse events that necessitate discontinuing therapy. For patients without these risk factors, quinolones may be a reasonable option.

4. Oguzturk H, Ozgur D, Turtay MG, Kayaalp C, Yilmaz S, Dogan M, Pamukcu E. Tramadol or paracetamol do not effect the diagnostic accuracy of acute abdominal pain with significant pain relief - a prospective, randomized, placebo controlled double blind study. Eur Rev Med Pharmacol Sci. 2012 Dec;16(14):1983-8. PMID: 23242726.

5. Schmieder G, Stankov G, Zerle G, Schinzel S, Brune K. Observer-blind study with metamizole versus tramadol and butylscopolamine in acute biliary colic pain. Arzneimittelforschung. 1993 Nov;43(11):1216-21. PMID: 8292068.

6. Turturro MA, Paris PM, Larkin GL. Tramadol versus hydrocodone-acetaminophen in acute musculoskeletal pain: a randomized, double-blind clinical trial. Ann Emerg Med. 1998 Aug;32(2):139-43. doi: 10.1016/s0196-0644(98)70127-1. PMID: 9701294.

7. Zeng C, Dubreuil M, LaRochelle MR, Lu N, Wei J, Choi HK, Lei G, Zhang Y. Association of Tramadol With All-Cause Mortality Among Patients With Osteoarthritis. JAMA. 2019 Mar 12;321(10):969-982. doi: 10.1001/jama.2019.1347. PMID: 30860559; PMCID: PMC6439672.

TRIMETHOPRIM-SULFAMETHOXAZOLE

I don't want to suggest TMP-Sulfa should never be used, but instead highlight that it can be high risk in **specific populations** like elderly patients or those with CKD. TMP-Sulfa has been shown to cause metabolic derangements like **hyponatremia, hypoglycemia,** and, most concerning, **hyperkalemia.** It can also cause dysfunction or injury of multiple organ systems, including the **liver** (drug-induced liver injury), **hematologic** (agranulocytosis, hemolytic anemia), and the **kidney** via an **AKI,** which is a problem in and of itself and a synergistic problem with the hyperkalemia noted above.

TMP-Sulfa is notorious as a causative agent in **multiple severe drug reaction syndromes**, like Stevens-Johnson syndrome (SJS), Toxic epidermal necrolysis (TEN), drug reaction with eosinophil syndrome (DRESS). It causes higher rates of **C. diff** than many other antibiotics and causes one of the worst interactions with warfarin. I avoid it in all elderly patients and choose other options if available for younger patients.

GABAPENTINOIDS

These are only indicated for purely **neuropathic pain** syndromes but are often prescribed **off-label** for indications that data suggests very limited or no efficacy (e.g., joint pain). Many patients on gabapentin complain of "brain fog." **Elderly adults are at the highest relative risk for adverse effects** like drowsiness, dizziness, falls, respiratory depression, confusion, and delirium, all of which increase the risk of accidents while driving. It is **renally-cleared**, so use extra caution in patients with CKD or AKI. There is an increased risk of overdose when combined with other sedating medications. There are also issues with **withdrawal symptoms** when discontinuing.

GLUCOCORTICOIDS (E.G., PREDNISONE)

Similar "indication creep" issues have been seen with glucocorticoids. Steroids are important medications and the first-line agent for many diseases. However, that doesn't mean they are wonderdrugs that can treat everything, nor are they risk-free. I regularly see clinicians prescribe steroids for everything from non-radicular back pain to cough, which the guidelines do not support.

The safety concerns of steroids are real, with most issues in **long-term use** like osteoporosis, **adrenal suppression**, hyperglycemia, and **Cushing's syndrome**. But don't forget even in short-term use, higher doses can cause sleep disturbances, mood disorder flares, mild immunosuppression, gastritis, GI bleeds, swelling, and elevation of WBC that can cloud clinical pictures if patients return later.[8] One study even found that short-term steroid use was associated with a higher rate of serious adverse events like **sepsis**, **DVT**, and **fractures**.[9] These risks and other steroid pearls are nicely summarized in a great *CoreIM Podcast*.[10]

DIPHENHYDRAMINE

Diphenhydramine is frequently prescribed for many conditions and is safe in many patients. However, some experts emphasize that the **side effect profile is terrible in elderly patients**, and the typical indications would all be better served by **newer-generation agents**. Safety concerns include the many **anti-cholinergic side effects** of drowsiness, confusion, urinary retention, tachycardia, nausea, and constipation. For this reason, it is listed on the Beers list of medications to avoid in elderly patients. The notes at the bottom of the page list an excellent podcast covering the risks and rationale for taking diphenhydramine out of your routine medication list.[11]

HYPERKALEMIA MEDICATIONS

Remember that **hyperkalemia** is one of the most dangerous electrolyte abnormalities. Several medications predictably raise the potassium level, so pay particular attention to this when prescribing the medications below:

- **ACE inhibitors**, like lisinopril.
- **ARBs**, like losartan.

8. "Association Between Oral Corticosteroid Bursts and Severe Adverse Events: A Nationwide Population-Based Cohort Study: Annals of Internal Medicine: Vol 173, No 5." Accessed July 24, 2023. https://www.acpjournals.org/doi/abs/10.7326/m20-0432.
9. Waljee A K, Rogers M A M, Lin P, Singal A G, Stein J D, Marks R M et al. Short term use of oral corticosteroids and related harms among adults in the United States: population based cohort study BMJ 2017; 357 :j1415 doi:10.1136/bmj.j1415
10. Core IM Podcast. "Steroids: 5 Pearls Segment," June 28, 2023. https://www.coreimpodcast.com/2023/06/28/steroid/.
11. "Diphenhydramine | FOAMcast." Accessed January 1, 2023. https://foamcast.org/tag/diphenhydramine/.

- **Potassium-sparing diuretics**, like spironolactone or triamterene.
- **Trimethoprim-sulfamethoxazole.**
- **Digoxin.**
- **Potassium supplements**, like potassium chloride.

Double-check the patient's last metabolic panel for potassium level and renal function when considering these medications. Avoid them in those with borderline-high potassium or those with significant CKD or AKI. Periodically recheck the patient's metabolic panel to monitor their potassium levels.

CARDIOLOGY MEDICATIONS

AMIODARONE

Long-term use of amiodarone is associated with several severe and potentially life-threatening risks. **Pulmonary toxicity** is a major concern, manifesting as pneumonitis or fibrosis. **Hepatotoxicity** is another risk that requires regular liver function monitoring. Amiodarone can also cause **thyroid dysfunction**, leading to either hypo- or hyperthyroidism due to its high iodine content. Long-term use may result in corneal deposits and optic neuropathy. Due to these risks, long-term use necessitates close and regular monitoring of pulmonary, hepatic, thyroid, and ocular function. It is class D in pregnancy. As detailed by Dr. Amal Mattu in this presentation, there are also risks in short-term use in the hospital.[12]

WARFARIN

This medication is notorious for its **countless interactions** with drugs and common foods like leafy green vegetables, after which the patient may have a subtherapeutic INR predisposing them to clotting or a supratherapeutic INR that might result in **catastrophic bleeding.** When possible, choose the newer oral anticoagulants without the interaction profile of warfarin. If your patient on warfarin needs any new prescription,

---

12. https://www.ucsfcme.com/2014/MEM14002/slides/10.MATTU_Tachycardia_Pitfalls.pdf

always double-check interactions on a reliable reference like UpToDate to see if it's safe.

DIGOXIN

In both the short and long term, digoxin can cause several adverse effects, particularly if dosing is not carefully managed given its notorious narrow therapeutic window. The most immediate risk is **digoxin toxicity,** which can occur if the dose is too high or if the patient has **kidney dysfunction.** Symptoms of toxicity include nausea, diarrhea, abdominal pain, **bradycardia,** and **arrhythmias like heart block.** Neurological effects include dizziness, confusion, and **visual disturbances** (e.g., seeing halos around lights or color distortion) can also occur. Immediate monitoring of blood levels and patient symptoms is essential to manage these risks effectively.

MENTAL HEALTH AND NEUROLOGICAL MEDICATIONS

BENZODIAZEPINES (E.G., LORAZEPAM, DIAZEPAM)

Patients often request these medications for the treatment of conditions like anxiety, but you should know the numerous safety concerns and consider alternatives first.

In short-term use, common side effects include **sedation, drowsiness, dizziness, and impaired coordination,** which can significantly affect a patient's ability to perform tasks like driving. Cognitive effects include **confusion, delirium, and memory impairment,** particularly in elderly patients. Respiratory depression can occur, especially when benzodiazepines are taken in high doses or in combination with other central nervous system depressants like alcohol or opioids.

Long-term use of benzodiazepines is associated with additional serious risks. One of the main concerns is the development of tolerance and physical dependence, leading to **withdrawal symptoms** when the medication is reduced or discontinued. Withdrawal symptoms can be severe, including potentially life-threatening **seizures and status epilepticus.** Long-term benzodiazepine use is associated with an increased risk of falls and fractures, particularly in older adults.

TRICYCLIC ANTIDEPRESSANTS (E.G., AMITRIPTYLINE)

These are considered "nonspecific drugs" given their effect on multiple neurotransmitters and receptors, resulting in potential adverse events like **serotonin syndrome, cardiovascular complications** (e.g., heart block, ventricular arrhythmias, sudden death), **anticholinergic effects, decreased seizure threshold,** anti-histamine effects, and sexual dysfunction. These medications have a high mortality in overdose.

FIRST-GENERATION ANTI-PSYCHOTICS (E.G., HALOPERIDOL, OLANZAPINE, RISPERIDONE)

First-generation antipsychotics pose several risks to patients. The most significant side effects include **extrapyramidal symptoms (EPS)** such as acute **dystonia** (painful muscle spasms), **akathisia** (severe restlessness), and **parkinsonism** (tremors and rigidity). Long-term use can lead to **tardive dyskinesia (TD)**, characterized by involuntary, repetitive movements, like tongue smacking, which can be irreversible. Cardiovascular risks like **QT prolongation** can result in serious arrhythmias.

Clozapine is an atypical antipsychotic used in the treatment of schizophrenia. It has a black box warning for the unique risks of **agranulocytosis with severe neutropenia,** lowering **seizure** threshold, and several **cardiovascular effects** (bradycardia, syncope, myocarditis, and myocarditis).

FIRST-GENERATION ANTI-EPILEPTIC MEDICATIONS

This class includes medications like carbamazepine, phenytoin, and valproate, which epileptologists still routinely prescribe. These meds have a high risk of **CNS depression, hepatotoxicity,** and **dermatologic emergencies** (e.g., Stevens-Johnson syndrome and DRESS syndrome). Consider these conditions anytime your patient on these medications presents with a rash. They are also highly **teratogenic**.

These medications require monitoring because of a narrow therapeutic window; you should double-check the patient's drug levels if they share **vague symptoms or report breakthrough seizures.** Interestingly, when levels are **too high**, it can paradoxically *decrease* the seizure threshold.

_____

IMMUNOSUPPRESSANTS AND BIOLOGICS

GENERAL CONSIDERATIONS

Immunosuppressants and biologic medications are now used in many specialties, including oncology for cancer treatment, gastroenterology for IBD management, rheumatology, and transplant surgery. There are many medications with varied mechanisms of action that are expanding every year, but recognize the following types of names that fit into this broad category of high-risk medications:

- Cyclosporine, cyclophosphamide, tacrolimus
- Cisplatin, carboplatin
- Rapamycin, bleomycin, doxorubicin
- Etanercept, abatacept
- Infliximab, rituximab, imatinib, dasatinib
- Methotrexate, azathioprine
- Paclitaxel, docetaxel
- Capecitabine, gemcitabine
- Vincristine, vinblastine

Whenever you manage a patient taking medications like this, remember the following risks that are common across most of them:

- **Severe infections** from bacteria *as well as* fungal and other opportunistic infections like tuberculosis.
- **Bone marrow suppression** and associated risks from neutropenia, anemia, and thrombocytopenia.
- **Teratogenicity**, and thus are high-risk in women of childbearing age.
- **Hepatotoxicity, nephrotoxicity, and cardiomyopathies.**
- **Malignancies,** like lymphoma and skin cancers.

IMMUNE CHECKPOINT INHIBITORS

These are a unique class of medications that has recently come into the spotlight as oncologists are increasingly prescribing them to treat cancer with great success. However, if you're following a patient who is taking one of these "-umab" medications (e.g., atezolizumab, pembrolizumab, and nivolumab), know that these are particularly high-risk medications with the broadest range of serious complications. The adverse effects broadly fall into **gland problems** like endocrinopathies and **solid organ inflammation and dysfunction.**

The **endocrinopathies** include the thyroid gland (thyroiditis), pituitary gland (hypopituitarism), adrenal gland (adrenal insufficiency), and pancreas (insulin-deficient diabetes).

The **solid organ inflammatory conditions** include the lungs (pneumonitis), colon (colitis), kidney (nephritis), brain (encephalitis), and heart (myocarditis).

Several of these are life-threatening, so whenever a patient on these medications reports new symptoms to you, take them very seriously and ask for help.

————

THE BETTER APPROACH

Recognizing high-risk medications and exercising caution when prescribing them is integral to safe patient care. If you find yourself considering any of the higher-risk medications, remember the actions to take from **habit six** in the prior chapter:

- Consider whether any **alternatives** would be a better option.
- **Ask for help** from a pharmacist or attending physician.
- **Inform your patient** of the medication's risks and use shared decision-making to make the final decision to prescribe.
- Give your patient good **discharge instructions**, explaining **when to stop** taking the medication.
- **Thoroughly document** your rationale and the conversation in your MDM.

Understanding medication hazards and safer alternatives will go a long way in helping you prevent iatrogenic harm.

CHAPTER 40

HIGH-RISK PATIENT POPULATIONS FOR MEDICATIONS

Knowing your patient's background medical information and tailoring your medication choice to their unique needs is critical. Let's review four of the most common patient populations that pose unique challenges for prescribers. We will also touch on symptom control for each population since it is the most common thing you'll need to treat.

PREGNANCY AND LACTATION

Double-check every medication you consider giving a pregnant or breastfeeding patient with a reliable reference like UpToDate. Some other good references include Brigg's Drugs in Pregnancy and Lactation, LactMed, and UpToDate. As a general rule, choose the lowest effective dose for the minimum duration.

A few notorious medications to avoid in pregnancy include **anti-epileptic medications**, most **anticoagulants**, **lithium**, **benzodiazepines**, certain **antibiotics** (sulfas, quinolones, tetracyclines, among others), **NSAIDs**, and **prochlorperazine**.

A prevalent pregnancy symptom is nausea, for which the first-line therapy is Diclegis (doxylamine with pyridoxine, aka vitamin B6). Second-line agents include options like diphenhydramine and metoclopramide. UpToDate has an excellent algorithm that summarizes the stepwise management approach.[1]

---

1. Smith, Judith. "Nausea and Vomiting of Pregnancy: Treatment and Outcome - UpToDate." Accessed December 29, 2022.

CKD AND ESRD

You'll need to double-check the safety and dosage of every medication you consider prescribing to patients with advanced CKD or ESRD. Avoiding nephrotoxic medications like NSAIDs is critical. Moreover, there are risks of decreased clearance of metabolites, so cross-check your reference to see if any potential prescription needs dose adjustment. If you have access to a pharmacist for questions, they are fantastic at guiding you in managing symptoms in those with ESRD and offering dose adjustment recommendations.

A stepwise ladder for pain control in ESRD is suggested in the article "...Pain management in patients with advanced kidney failure." Dr. Sara Davison recommends **acetaminophen** (max 2-3g daily), then consider a **topical NSAID** like Voltaren gel if the pain is localized to one joint. If a patient is entirely anuric, sometimes other NSAIDs can be considered. Opiates should be avoided when possible in patients on dialysis, as they are associated with altered mental status, increased rate of falls and fractures, and higher mortality.[2,3]

CIRRHOSIS

The liver is the other key organ responsible for processing many medications. For those with impaired liver function, you'll need to double-check every potential prescription to see if it is hepatically cleared.

In patients with cirrhosis, it is best to avoid **acetaminophen** if they are actively drinking and have the potential for associated liver injury. If they are not drinking and don't have any evidence of acute liver injury / LFT derangement, you can consider acetaminophen at a reduced dose with a max of 2g/day for short-term use. **NSAIDs** are also high risk, given the increased bleeding risk in cirrhotic patients.

Opioids are also high risk because they can precipitate hepatic encephalopathy and hospitalization. Thus they should be avoided if possible in patients with cirrhosis, especially those with portal

2. Ishida, Julie. *Clinical Journal of the American Society of Nephrology* 13(5):p 746-753, May 2018. | DOI: 10.2215/CJN.09910917
3. Kimmel PL, Fwu CW, Abbott KC, Eggers AW, Kline PP, Eggers PW. Opioid Prescription, Morbidity, and Mortality in United States Dialysis Patients. J Am Soc Nephrol. 2017 Dec;28(12):3658-3670. doi: 10.1681/ASN.2017010098. Epub 2017 Sep 21. PMID: 28935654; PMCID: PMC5698071.

hypertension and encephalopathy. For further reading, check out this reference article at the bottom of this page.[4]

ELDERLY PATIENTS

Elderly patients frequently have long lists of home medications, making them at much higher risk for drug interactions. Unfortunately, they often don't remember what they're taking. Ask the family to take a picture and send you the medications they are actually taking.

It's also helpful to study the Beers List of high-risk medications in elderly patients.[5] Here are a few of the classes of medicines included in the list:

- Medications with **anticholinergic side effects**, like anti-histamines, antispasmodics, TCAs, and many other medications. Elderly patients are particularly prone to anticholinergic side effects, like confusion, dry mouth, urinary retention, constipation, and more.
- Cardiovascular medications can drop blood pressure or cause dizziness (and therefore falls), like **alpha blockers, calcium channel blockers, and antiarrhythmics.**
- Medications that can cause hyperkalemia, especially in elderly patients with impaired renal function, like **spironolactone, lisinopril, and trimethoprim-sulfamethoxazole (TMP-Sulfa).**
- **Benzodiazepines**, the classic teaching is that giving benzodiazepines to older adults can have a paradoxical effect of increased agitation and risk of delirium and falls.
- **NSAIDs** with their many risks for elderly patients.
- **Muscle relaxants** with risk of sedation and falls.

Knowing which patients are at high risk for medication adverse events is a key step in responsible prescribing. If you've identified your patient is high-risk, it's time to stop and think. Double-check the information on

4. Chandok N, Watt KD. Pain management in the cirrhotic patient: the clinical challenge. Mayo Clin Proc. 2010 May;85(5):451-8. doi: 10.4065/mcp.2009.0534. Epub 2010 Mar 31. PMID: 20357277; PMCID: PMC2861975.
5. "Geriatrics Care | Beer's Criteria Authors." Accessed December 31, 2022. https:// geriatricscareonline.org/.

reliable resources or ask someone more experienced for help. Last, use shared decision-making and document well.

CHAPTER 41
PAIN MEDICATIONS AND PITFALLS

PAIN WILL BE the most common symptom for which patients request medication. You'll soon experience how stressful these situations can be. Imagine a grown adult sitting before you, verbally escalating as they demand pain pills that you don't feel are in their best interest.

Pain management is a challenging topic that requires understanding the different medications available and the risks/benefits of each. This chapter will review the options and strategies to manage these stressful situations.

————

ACETAMINOPHEN:

- What is the standard dosage, daily max, and contraindications for acetaminophen?
- If you are concerned about APAP toxicity because your patient accidentally took too much or took it without realizing a contraindication exists, what treatment is available to prevent toxicity?

Acetaminophen is a safe medication for pain control for most patients. The max dosage is **3-4g/day in normal patients**.

Avoid acetaminophen if you see evidence of acute liver injury/LFT elevation or decompensated cirrhosis. In those with stable cirrhosis, or low body weight (<50kg), you can still give APAP, but the max dosage should be reduced to 2 grams daily.[1]

Treatment for APAP toxicity is **N-acetyl cysteine (NAC)**. There are a few scenarios that can result in APAP toxicity[2]:

- **A single large ingestion:** For example, in a suicide attempt. The Rumack-Matthew Nomogram is used in combination with a serum APAP level to determine if NAC is required.
- **Repeated dosing over the recommended amount:** For example, in a patient with uncontrolled pain who takes too much Tylenol. Toxicity occurs with doses over 6g per 24-hour period for two days.
- **Therapeutic dosing in the setting of acute liver injury:** For example, in a patient with elevated LFTs from binging alcohol who took 4g of Tylenol to treat their heartburn.

In all of these situations, the **poison control center** (800-222-1222) is a free and fantastic resource for immediate guidance for these patients.

NSAIDS (IBUPROFEN, NAPROXEN, KETOROLAC):

- What are the three major risks of the NSAID class of medications?
- How can you minimize those risks in a patient you think would benefit from NSAIDs?

NSAIDs are commonly used medications but be mindful of the significant risks of the NSAID class of medications, which include but are not limited to the following:

Risks after single ingestion: Kidney injury, platelet dysfunction, and increased risk of bleeding. Thus, these should be avoided in GI bleeding and after head injuries.

1. Imani F, Motavaf M, Safari S, Alavian SM. The therapeutic use of analgesics in patients with liver cirrhosis: a literature review and evidence-based recommendations. Hepat Mon. 2014 Oct 11;14(10):e23539. doi: 10.5812/hepatmon.23539. PMID: 25477978; PMCID: PMC4250965.

2. Heard MD, Kennon. "Acetaminophen (Paracetamol) Poisoning in Adults: Treatment - UpToDate," n.d. Accessed December 29, 2022.

Risks after longer-term use: *GI complications* (peptic ulcer disease, GI bleeding), *cardiovascular complications* (HTN, myocardial infarction, worsening of heart failure, and stroke), and *renal complications* (AKI, CKD, and electrolyte abnormalities).[3]

If patients are otherwise young and healthy, short courses of NSAIDs are reasonable options. However, avoid longer courses in most patients and any amount in high-risk populations.

How to minimize the risks of NSAIDs? Use topical therapy (Voltaren gel) when able, and use the shortest possible course (days>weeks) for all others.

_____

MISC NON-OPIATES

- **Lidoderm patch** - 4% is over-the-counter, and 5% is by prescription. These can work surprisingly well for some conditions, like rib fractures.
- **Muscle relaxants**, like methocarbamol (Robaxin), can work well for some patients but should be avoided in elderly patients (Beer's List) due to dizziness, falls, and sedation risks. Driving and operating machinery should also be avoided.
- **Gabapentinoids** (gabapentin and pregabalin) are often used to treat neuropathic pain and require slow titration up and down, given the risk for withdrawal. There are also risks of drowsiness, respiratory depression, and confusion. These side effects are worsened by renal dysfunction or when combined with other CNS-suppressive medications.

_____

OPIOIDS

- What are the most commonly used opioid medications and their standard dosing?

_____

3. Solomon MD, Daniel. "Nonselective NSAIDs: Overview of Adverse Effects - UpToDate," n.d. Accessed December 29, 2022.

- What are the contraindications to prescribing opioids and patient populations that should be used with caution?
- What are the risks and side effects of opiate medications?
- What are the signs and symptoms of opiate toxicity, and what is the treatment?
- What are the signs and symptoms of opiate withdrawal?

Here are the most commonly used opioid medications in acute care and their dosing:

- **Hydrocodone-acetaminophen (Norco)** — 5mg PO given every 4-6 hours. A common oral pain medication.
- **Oxycodone +/- acetaminophen (Percocet)** — 5mg PO q4-6 hours. Another common oral pain medication. Oxycodone is stronger than hydrocodone.
- **Morphine** — 0.1mg/kg/dose with a typical max of 4mg IV/IM. Be mindful that morphine causes a histamine release and thus can more potently drop blood pressure than alternatives.
- **Fentanyl** — 50 - 100 mcg IV/IM every 1 to 2 hours. It is short-acting and useful for procedures.
- **Hydromorphone (Dilaudid)** — 0.2-1mg IV every 2-3 hours. This is the strongest opiate. Avoid in those who are opiate naive, given concern for respiratory depression.

Avoid opiates in liver failure, renal failure, patients at risk for respiratory depression (especially chronic hypercapnia like COPD), and elderly patients (Beer's list).

All opiates are **sedating**, so patients should be advised not to drive or operate machinery. The patient's respiratory status and vital signs should be monitored when given via the IV route.

Other adverse side effects of opiates include **constipation**, nausea, **respiratory depression**, **hypotension**, **dependence**, and **opioid hyperalgesia syndrome**, in which the patient's perception of pain gets worse after getting accustomed to opiates.[4]

It is best practice to consider each patient's risk for addiction. This could be based on your clinical gestalt, or if you prefer a more objective

4. Benyamin R, Trescot AM, Datta S, Buenaventura R, Adlaka R, Sehgal N, Glaser SE, Vallejo R. Opioid complications and side effects. Pain Physician. 2008 Mar;11(2 Suppl):S105-20. PMID: 18443635.

measure, you can try a scoring system like the **Opioid Risk Tool (ORT)** on MD-Calc.

BRINGING IT ALL TOGETHER

For patients presenting with a complaint of pain, the best practice is to optimize as much of a **non-opiate multimodal pain control regimen first** and only consider opiates on a limited basis when appropriate after that. Try a combination of acetaminophen, Voltaren gel, and a lidocaine patch for decent pain control with minimal risks. Consider adding a muscle relaxant next for young and healthy patients with musculoskeletal pain.

For patients with acute severe pain, like from a fracture, **it is reasonable to add a short course of an opiate** after calculating their ORT score. If they score high risk for addiction, be sure to have a frank discussion with them about the risks and involve a family member to help monitor for appropriate use.

Remember that your state regulations may clarify acceptable prescribing practices. In Washington state, for example, the WA Health Care Authority (HCA) policy limits the quantity of opioids that can be prescribed to opiate naïve patients for non-cancer pain. The limits are[5]:

- No more than 18 doses (**approximately a 3-day supply**) for patients aged 20 or younger.
- No more than 42 doses (**approximately a 7-day supply**) for patients aged 21 or older.

For more perspectives on this topic of symptom control medications, check out other guides shared freely online:

- For a formal guide, check out the "SAEM Acute Pain Control Guide."[6]

---

5. https://www.hca.wa.gov/billers-providers-partners/program-information-providers/opioids
6. Default. "Acute Pain Control." Accessed March 6, 2023. https://www.saem.org/about-saem/academies-interest-groups-affiliates2/cdem/for-students/online-education/m3-curriculum/group-acute-pain-control/acute-pain-control.

- For popular informal guides, search for "Reddit Conaanaa's Guides for Noobs" in pain control. He also has guides on bowel regiments, electrolyte replacement, and more that are fun reads.

CHAPTER 42
ANTIBIOTICS IN CLINICAL PRACTICE

"I am almost done with PA school and I still don't feel like I am anywhere near understanding antibiotics. I was overwhelmed by all the information shared in our school's Powerpoints, and I don't feel like I've retained anything. I find myself just nodding my head whenever my preceptor talks about antibiotic choice without truly understanding why. Help!"

PA STUDENT, 2022

ANTIBIOTIC THERAPY IS another topic that many new graduates find challenging. The antibiotic lectures we heard in grad school do not always present the information in the same way they come up in practice.

How does it come up in clinical practice? There are a few common situations. You might be asking yourself these questions — or they might be asked by your attending/pharmacist/consultant:

- "You have a confirmed **diagnosis** (e.g., acute appendicitis), so what is the **first-line antibiotic**?"
- "How will you cover [gram-negatives] for this patient with [sepsis] and a suspected [abdominal source]?" In other words, you need to know *empiric* **coverage** based on each *class of bacteria* when you don't have a definitive diagnosis.

- "So you are considering treatment with [ciprofloxacin+flagyl] —
  are there any concerns about this choice with this patient?" In
  other words, you need to consider the *patient factors* and the
  antibiotic class features to know if it is the right choice for this
  patient. If you determine that the first-line agent is inappropriate
  for this patient, what is the second-line agent?

These questions will encompass 95% of what you'll have to solve in
clinical practice. In this chapter, I will share the fundamentals so that you
can confidently answer these questions and more.

———

DX —> BUG —> DRUG

This is the most common situation you will encounter. From the starting
point, "I think the patient is suffering from diagnosis X," you must figure
out the best antibiotic to treat them using a four-step approach.

1. What is the suspected diagnosis?
2. Based on the Dx, what are the most likely bacteria?
3. Based on the bacteria, what is the best antibiotic choice?
4. Review the patient's background information and consider the
   drug's interactions and adverse effects to ensure it is the right
   choice for this patient.

Your local antibiogram is the best way to answer question (3), but we
will cover some general rules of thumb below. Eventually, you can skip
step (2), but you should try to learn and internalize this knowledge during
your first year. The new graduates who never learn what they are trying to
treat will be prone to errors when patients present atypically or with an
unclear clinical picture.

Okay, let's use cellulitis as an example to illustrate this section on a
diagnosis-driven approach. We divide the diagnosis of cellulitis into
purulent cellulitis versus *non-purulent* cellulitis because each of these has
different culprit bacteria and, therefore, different treatment needs.

Whenever you see purulence, such as in abscesses or the "wet" draining cellulitis, you should think Staph aureus (and MRSA) is the likely cause. The best available antibiotics for staph/MRSA coverage (*which still might not be great depending on where you live*) include oral options TMP-Sulfa, clindamycin, doxycycline, and linezolid (very expensive). The most common IV option for MRSA is vancomycin.

Non-purulent cellulitis, on the other hand, is most commonly caused by streptococcus species, which are better treated by cephalosporins like cephalexin, cefadroxil, or clindamycin for oral options, and ceftriaxone or cefazolin for IV options.

Here are some more common clinical situations, again organized as *diagnosis —> bugs —> antibiotic options*. Challenge yourself by getting a sheet of paper and answering what you think are the likely bacterial culprits and antibiotics you'd choose for each of the following:

- Throat and oral infections, like bacterial tonsillitis.
- Lung infections, like pneumonia.
- Urinary tract infections, like cystitis.
- GI infections, like diverticulitis.

Throat and oral infections, like bacterial tonsillitis—> streptococcus pyogenes (GAS) —> penicillin, amoxicillin, and clindamycin. A complicated infection like a deep space infection or abscess will need anaerobic coverage (discussed below) with something like amoxicillin-clavulanate.

Lung infections like pneumonia —> "typical" bacterial infections like streptococcus pneumoniae, klebsiella, and haemophilus influenzae have the treatment options of beta-lactams or respiratory fluoroquinolones. The "atypical" bacteria like mycoplasma pneumoniae, legionella, and chlamydia pneumoniae have first-line treatment options of a macrolide (azithromycin) or doxycycline. Second-line treatment options include respiratory fluoroquinolones.

Urinary tract infections like cystitis and pyelonephritis —> gram-negative infections like E.coli —> first-line agents include cephalosporins like cefadroxil/cephalexin and nitrofurantoin. Second-

242

line considerations are TMP-sulfa, fosfomycin, and fluoroquinolones. Pyelonephritis should not be treated with cefadroxil or nitrofurantoin. Ceftriaxone is the most commonly used IV option.

GI infections like diverticulitis or appendicitis —> gram-negative and anaerobic coverage —> Conditions like uncomplicated diverticulitis, when requiring antibiotics, can be treated orally with agents like amoxicillin-clavulanate or PO ciprofloxacin+metronidazole. The most commonly used IV option is ceftriaxone + metronidazole.

BUG CLASS —> EXAMPLE BUGS —> DRUGS

Consultants or supervising physicians often comment from the reference point of bacteria class instead of the specific diagnosis to help guide antibiotic choice. This is especially true when you don't have a definitive diagnosis and are considering empiric coverage.

The following are the most common types of requests you'll hear from your attendings and consultants. Challenge yourself by guessing the clinical situation these might occur, what bacteria are the typical culprits, and what antibiotic options you'd choose to manage these:

- "We need **gram-positive** coverage."
- "Do you have **gram-negative** coverage?"
- "Let's add **atypical** coverage."
- "Please add **anaerobic** coverage."
- "Make sure the antibiotic has **pseudomonas** coverage."

"We need *gram-positive coverage*," ... which generally refers to **staph and strep** coverage. This would be needed to treat cellulitis, osteomyelitis under an ulcer, or pneumonia that developed after influenza (classically caused by staph). Options include cephalexin + TMP-Sulfa/doxycycline, clindamycin, linezolid for oral coverage, and vancomycin or linezolid for IV coverage.

"We need *gram-negative coverage*," ... aka **E. coli** coverage (as well as klebsiella, etc.), which might be needed to treat something like an intra-abdominal infection or a UTI. Options for UTI tx include cephalosporins, amoxicillin-clavulanate, TMP-sulfa, and fluoroquinolones for oral coverage, and ceftriaxone for IV coverage.

"We need *atypical coverage"* ... for treatment of something like community-acquired pneumonia with bilateral lung findings. Options include azithromycin and doxycycline for both oral and IV coverage. Fluoroquinolones also have typical and atypical coverage, but we avoid prescribing them when able and prefer to get atypical coverage from alternative means.

"We need *anaerobic coverage"* ... for treatment of something like an ENT abscess, intra-abdominal abscess, or a wound infected from an animal bite —> Options include amoxicillin-clavulanate, metronidazole for oral coverage, ampicillin/sulbactam (Unasyn), piperacillin/tazobactam (Zosyn), and metronidazole for IV coverage.

"We need *pseudomonas coverage"* ... for treatment of something like a positive culture growing pseudomonas, neutropenic fever, or diabetic foot osteomyelitis —> The only oral options currently are the fluoroquinolones ciprofloxacin or levofloxacin (<u>NOT</u> moxifloxacin), and even these have limited efficacy related to infection location and regional resistance. For IV coverage, cefepime, piperacillin/tazobactam, meropenem, or fluoroquinolones are all options.

ANTIBIOTIC CLASS CONSIDERATIONS

At this point of the clinical encounter, you have a specific antibiotic in mind for treating your patient, but you can't stop there. You need to consider the patient factors and the antibiotic features to ensure they are a good match with no contraindications.

Another way of framing this is — what comes to the minds of practicing clinicians when they consider an antibiotic? What are the unique features of the following antibiotic classes? Quiz yourself by writing what comes to your mind for each of the following classes of antibiotics.

Penicillins — This class of antibiotics is well-tolerated but is losing efficacy to bacterial resistance. They are most commonly used for gram-positive coverage, with some limited coverage of gram-negative organisms. If your antibiogram still lists them as first-line therapy, great — use them! They have an excellent safety profile.

You will hear all the time, "I can't take penicillins — my mother thought I had a [insert vague description of a possible allergic reaction] as an infant" ... these are seldom true allergies. To deal with these situations, look up the cross-reactivity tables with cephalosporins and consider test doses of antibiotics. If the patient is truly pen-allergic, as long as it wasn't an anaphylactic allergy, you can still safely give a cephalosporin if they don't share the same side chain (i.e., 3rd generation cephalosporin is usually okay).

Amoxicillin-clavulanate — While not a *class* of antibiotics, it is considered a unique and strong antibiotic that stands out from the rest of the penicillin class. It is still first-line for many specific indications like sinusitis, AOM in adults, animal bites, diverticulitis, and more. It treats anaerobes in addition to its gram-positive and negative coverage. It requires counseling patients on the risk of diarrhea and C. diff, and you can consider recommending probiotics.

Cephalosporins — This is a workhorse class of antibiotics. They are widely used because of how well they work, how well-tolerated they are, and because they don't have as many serious adverse reactions as the other classes. If you see a cephalosporin as a treatment option, it's often a great choice. First-generation cephalosporins like cephalexin and cefazolin (Ancef) predominantly provide gram-positive coverage with a small amount of gram-negative coverage and, thus are good choices for things like non-purulent cellulitis. Remember that cephalexin requires QID dosing to maintain therapeutic levels throughout the day. Cefadroxil is another first-generation agent that some prefer given BID dosing. As you go up in generations, the third-generation cephalosporins like ceftriaxone add in more gram-negative coverage but lose some gram-positive coverage. Fourth-generation cephalosporins like cefepime add in pseudomonas coverage.

Fluoroquinolones (like levofloxacin or ciprofloxacin)— We won't belabor the points discussed earlier. Quinolone coverage includes predominantly gram-negative infections, including urinary and respiratory tract infections. Suppose you see multiple treatment options for a given indication (e.g., UTI). In that case, you should avoid quinolones because of the numerous adverse events that can result in patient harm.

Sulfonamides (TMP-Sulfa) — We won't repeat the content about TMP-Sulfa in the prior section. Beware of prescribing TMP-Sulfa in many patient populations. In otherwise young and healthy patients without other good options, sulfa antibiotics are still routinely used in practice. A good example would be patients who use IV drugs presenting with purulent cellulitis given the high rates of MRSA.

Tetracyclines (doxycycline) — Doxycycline is a wonderful antibiotic with many indications covering gram-positive and gram-negative bacteria, including skin infections, lungs, tick-borne illnesses, and many others. It is generally well-tolerated and, as a result, is a commonly prescribed antibiotic. It does have the risk of photosensitivity (counsel patients to avoid sunburns) and discoloring teeth in children and thus should be avoided in pediatrics and pregnancy.

Macrolides (azithromycin) — Macrolides like azithromycin, historically speaking, were widely prescribed and often for inappropriate indications. As a result, we now have significant resistance. They are well-tolerated and still used as an adjunct treatment for respiratory tract infections like atypical pneumonia or as a second-line agent for other infections in penicillin-allergic patients.

Glycopeptides (vancomycin) — Vancomycin is the hospital's workhouse gram-positive and MRSA agent. Remember that oral vancomycin *does not get absorbed systemically*, so you can't use it to treat outpatient MRSA skin infections (but you can use it to treat C. diff colitis by oral route). IV vancomycin is bacteriostatic, not bactericidal. This is relevant in patients with severe sepsis, for whom it's recommended to start the *other* antibiotic first if only one IV is available.

The following are **heavy-duty, restricted, or cost-prohibitive antibiotics you probably should not be ordering as a new graduate** without involvement by an attending physician or pharmacist: Cefepime, Ceftazidime, Meropenem, Imipenem, Ertapenem, Aztreonam, Linezolid, Amphotericin B.

PATIENT FACTORS

The last step in finalizing the best choice of antibiotic is considering the patient factors that significantly impact your decision-making. A common and illustrative example is seen with "culture callbacks," in which positive urine or blood cultures are routed to you on shift, even if it isn't your patient. The nurse might come up to you and say, "Dr. Martin's patient had a urine culture positive for E. coli that is sensitive to ciprofloxacin — can you give me a verbal order, and I will call it in?" The correct response is, "Let me review the chart first."

It is critical to assess all of the following background information for every patient you are considering antibiotics:

- **Age** — Certain antibiotics are high risk and contraindicated in children (doxycycline), while others are high risk in elderly patients (TMP-sulfamethoxazole).
- **Sex** — If you have a female patient of childbearing age, you must assess for pregnancy and breastfeeding status. For males treated for UTIs, assess for any signs or symptoms suggestive of prostatitis, for which only certain antibiotics have good prostate penetration.
- **PMH** — Do they have CKD, and what was their last GFR/creatinine clearance? Do they have cirrhosis? If either is present, check if that organ clears the antibiotic. If so, you should find an alternative or dose adjust using their creatinine clearance (preferred over GFR).
- **Other medications** — Always review their background medications and specifically ask about warfarin use, which interacts with almost everything.
- **Medication allergies** — This is an obvious point for review.

247

- **Clinical presentation** — What are their signs and symptoms? Treatment would vary if it's an upper versus lower urinary tract infection. What if they don't have any symptoms at all? Some positive urine cultures reflect *asymptomatic* bacteriuria, which does not require treatment in many people.[1] Exceptions that would require treatment regardless of symptoms include pregnant women, those who cannot provide any history (non-verbal), or those near surgery. Some say non-verbal patients should usually only receive treatment if they show systemic signs of illness (elevated serum WBC, fever, SIRS criteria, etc), but this is an area of debate.

MATERIALS FOR A DEEPER DIVE

If you will be prescribing antibiotics regularly, I recommend you dive deeper than the basics I have reviewed in this chapter. These are the best resources I've encountered to help you do so.

(1) Dx —> Bugs —> Drugs

- FirstLine App (integrates local antibiogram if your hospital system is affiliated)
- UpToDate
- "Antibiotics by Diagnosis - WikEM." https://wikem.org/wiki/Antibiotics_by_diagnosis.

(2) Bug class and organism —> Drugs

- *Great Youtube video: Antibiotic Coverage Made Easy | | USMLE | COMLEX*, 2019. https://www.youtube.com/watch?v=VTp86YN6diI.

1. Givler DN, Givler A. Asymptomatic Bacteriuria. [Updated 2023 Jul 17]. In: StatPearls [Internet]. Treasure Island (FL): StatPearls Publishing; 2024 Jan-. Available from: https://www.ncbi.nlm.nih.gov/books/NBK441848/

- https://www.idstewardship.com/bugs-drugs-study-table-pharmacy-school-exam/
- https://medfools.com/downloads/Bacteria.pdf
- https://www.wikem.org/wiki/Microbiology_(Main)

(3) Drug class —> Gram stain and bug coverage

- *Famous Youtube video: The Antibiotic Ladder Revisited: Anti-Infective Therapy Part 2*, 2019. https://www.youtube.com/watch?v=XXI0CtzrDv4.
- *Antibiotics Primer,* reboot Curbsiders Epp 284 (Podcast App)
- *Antibiotic Classes in 7 Minutes..* 2019. https://www.youtube.com/watch?v=gqoqexfqoBM.
- "Antibiotics Review." https://errolozdalga.com/medicine/pages/OtherPages/AntibioticReview.ChanuRhee.html — Fantastic reference that goes into much more depth and specifics than I did above.

(4) Good on-shift references:

- FirstLine App
- EMRA Abx guide
- Sanford guide
- UpToDate

CHAPTER 43
LIFE-SAVING MEDICATION REFERENCE

REGARDLESS OF WHAT setting you will be working in, there will always be the possibility for a patient to decompensate in front of you. Having a high-quality reference for the most common "emergency medications" will serve you well. **Dr. Sarah Foohey** (@SarahFoohey, and website First10EM.com) has made a fantastic reference and has graciously allowed me to share them with you here. Consider printing this out or saving it to your phone. On her website, you can check out the other infographics she has made.[1]

---

1. Foohey, Sarah. "Foohey's Figures - First10EM." Accessed December 29, 2022. https://first10em.com/fooheysfigures/.

MUST KNOW MEDS

Arrest
Defib 200J
Epi 1mg IV
Amiodarone 300mg then 150mg IV
Mg 2g IV (for VT/Torsades)
HCO3 2 amp IV Bolus
Calcium Gluconate 1 amp
Refractory VF: Esmolol 500mcg/kg IV bolus then 50mcg/kg/min + DSD.

Tachycardia
Cardioversion (Sync) 100, 150, 200J
Adenosine 6mg, then 12mg IV
Metoprolol 5mg IV, then 25mg PO
Diltiazem 10-20mg IV, then 120mg PO
Verapamil 2.5-10mg IV
Amiodarone 150mg over 10min
Procainamide 20mg/min then 1mg/min
Ottawa Protocol: Procainamide 1g/1hr.
Digoxin 0.25mg (or 0.125mg) IV, can repeat in 15m

Bradycardia
Atropine 1mg. Repeat up to 3mg.
Epinephrine 2-10mcg/min
Dopamine 2-20mcg/kg/min
Isopril 2-10mcg/min. 0.01-0.05mcg/kg/min.
Pacing: Start at 60.

Pressors & Inotropes
Levophed 2-20mcg/min
  0.05-2mcg/kg/min
Epinephrine 2-20mcg/min
  0.05-0.5mcg/kg/min
Vasopressin 0.04U/min, 1-5mg/hr
Dobutamine 2-20mcg/kg/min
~~Dopamine 2-20mcg/kg/min~~
HCO3 infusion 150mEq (3amps) in 1L D5W at 200cc/hr (remove 150cc from bag 1st)
PUSH Phenyl: 50-200mcg q2m (1mL of 10mg/mL in 100mL =100mcg/mL)

Sepsis: NE then Vaso
Cardiogenic: NE then low Dobutamine

Hypertension
Labetalol 20mg IV q10min. 0.5-2mg/min.
Esmolol 500mcg/kg/min bolus. 50mcg/kg/min.
Nitroprusside 0.25-3mcg/kg/min
Enalaprit 1.25mg IV
Hydralazine 10-20mg IV q30min (Peds: 0.5mg/kg)
Nicardipine 5mg/hr
Phentolamine 2.5-15mg IV (if ? cocaine/pheo)

Nitro 0.4mg SL q5min (0.4mg = 400mcg q5min w 60% uptake = 48mcg/min). Patch 0.4, 0.6, 1.2mg
Nitro 50-100-200mcg/min. 0.2-0.4mcg/kg/min.
Caution: Viagra/Cialis, Inf MI, low BP, AS, Pulm HTN

ACPE (HTN + SOB): Nitro, Enalaprit, Nitroprusside
Dissection: HR<60, BP<110. Labetalol, Nitroprusside
Neuro: Labetalol, Hydralazine. AVOID nitrogly/pruss.
Eclampsia: Mg, Labetalol, Hydralazine

MI
Heparin 60U/kg (ex: 4000U), 15U/kg/hr
ASA 160mg PO
Ticagrelor 180mg PO, Plavix 300mg PO
Nitro 0.4mg SL

Tenecteplase (TNK) IV bolus over 5sec. Half dose if age 76+.
<60kg: 30mg
60-70kg: 35mg
70-80kg: 40mg
80-90kg: 45mg
>90kg: 50mg

NSTEMI: Fondaparinox 2.5mg SC daily

HyperK
Calcium gluconate 1-2 amp
Insulin 5-10U IV (5 if CKD)
D50W 1-2 amp IV
Ventolin 4-8 puffs
Lasix 40-80mg IV (if V overload)
IV RL 1 bolus (if hypoV, avoid NS)
HCO3 1-2 amp or inf (if HCO3 <20)
Kayexelate 15-30g (in 30mL Lactul)
Digibind 10-20vials if Dig Tox

Seizures
Lorazepam 0.1mg/kg IM/IN/IV/PR. 2-4mg. 3m onset.
Midazolam 0.2mg/kg IM/IN/IV. 5-10mg. 30s.
Diazepam 0.2mg/kg IV. 5-10mg IV. 0.5mg/kg PR.

Fosphenytoin 20mg/kg IV/IM. Max 1.5g.
Phenytoin 20mg/kg IV. Max 1.5g. Avoid if ?Tox. 10m.
Phenobarb 20mg/kg IV. Max 1 g. Then intubate.
Valproate 20-40mg/kg IV (may not be available PO)
Levetiracetam 40-60mg/kg IV (Keppra; may not have)
Ketamine 0.5-3mg/kg IV then 0.3-4mg/kg/hr
Propofol 2-5mg/kg then 2-10mg/kg/hr (50-80ug/kg/m)

? Gluc, Na, Isoniazid (Pyridoxine 70mg/kg up to 5g),
Eclampsia (Mg 4-6g IV, 1-2g/hr), Thiamine (?EtOH wd)

Stroke
Alteplase 0.9mg/kg. 10% bolus, 90% over 1hr.
Mild TIA or mod-severe stroke (no lysis)*:
ASA 162-325mg PO daily
High risk TIA or minor stroke, Dual APT*:
ASA 160-325mg chewed then 81 daily
Plavix 300mg PO then 75mg daily x 21d
*Guidelines differ if AFib/anticoagulated.

High ICP (inc. DKA)
Mannitol 1-1.5g/kg over 20min (Or 5mL/kg)
Adult: 100g (500mL bag). Kids: 250mL.

3% NS 3mL/kg over 3min. Range: 3-10mL/kg
Adult: 250mL

Intubation
+/- Fentanyl 3mcg/kg pre-treat if neuro
Etomidate 0.3mg/kg IV
Propofol 1-2mg/kg IV
Ketamine 1-2mg/kg IV.
Midazolam 0.1-0.3mg/kg IV
Rocuronium 1.2-1.6mg/kg IV
Succinylcholine 1-2mg/kg IV
If shock: half induction, N/high paralytic
If brady: atropine 0.02mg/kg IV (age<1)
DSI: Ketamine 1mg/kg, 0.5mg/kg PRN until dissociated; while pre-oxygenating.

Awake Intubation
Glycopyrrolate 0.2mg IV, Zofran 4mg
Ketamine 10-20mg q30s (0.1-0.3mg/kg)
or: Midazolam 0.25-1mg (0.2mg/kg), Fentanyl 25-50mcg
Lidocaine 10mL of 4% spray, 5% ointment
Steps 1&3: Spray 4% aqueous lidocaine w atomizer
Step 2: "Melt" 5% ointment lidocaine off tongue dep.

Post Intubation IV Sedation
Fentanyl 2mcg/kg, 0.5-2mcg/kg/hr. 0-250mcg/hr
Propofol 0.5mg/kg, 1mg/kg/hr (0-200), 5-50mcg/kg/min
Ketamine 1mg/kg then 0.5-4mg/kg/hr
Midazolam 0.05-0.2mg/kg, 0.05-2mg/kr/hr, 0-20mg/hr,
  1-24mcg/kg/min.

Hyponatremia
3% NS 2mL/kg (100-150mL) over 10min.
Repeat x 1 in 10 minutes. Make SL/NPO.
Or: 1 amp NaHCO3 over 5min.

UO >100mL/hr + urine osmol <100:
DDAVP 1mcg IV

Vent Settings
VT 6-8mL/kg IBW
RR 16 (10 if asthma/COPD), IFR 60L/min
PEEP 5 (0 if asthma/COPD), FiO2 40%+

Anaphylaxis
Epi 0.5mg IM q5 x 3 1:1000 (0.01mg/kg)
Epi 3mL/5mL Neb (<10kg, >10kg))
Epi 2-20mcg/min IV
+ Glucagon 1mg IV/IM if on B-blocker
Benadryl 50mg PO/IV (1mg/kg)
Ranitidine 50mg IV (1mg/kg)
Cetirizine 2.5/5/10mg (<2,2-5,>5yr)
Methylprednisone 125mg IV (1mg/kg)
Prednisone 50mg PO (1-2mg/kg)
Dexamethasone 0.6mg/kg PO (peds)

HAE: Ecallantide 30mg SC, Berinert 20U/kg IV, Icatibant 30mc SC. Or: FFP.

Croup
Dex 0.6mg/kg PO
Epi Neb 3mL/5mL (</>10kg)

Asthma/COPD
Ventolin 2.5/5mg Neb (</>20kg), 4-8 puffs
Atrovent 250/500mcg Neb, 4-8 puffs
Mg 2g IV over 30min (50mg/kg)
Steroid, Epi - see anaphylaxis (Dex: 0.3-0.6mg/kg)
Ventolin 7.5mcg/kg IV bolus, 1-10mcg/kg/min infusion

Rx: Dex 0.3mg/kg x 1, Ventolin 100mcg 4q4hr PRN
Alvesco MDI 200mcg 1 puff (6-11), 2 puffs (>12) OD
Flovent MDI 125mcg BID (can use in <6yr)

BiPap Settings
COPD 8 insp + 3 exp
CHF 10 insp + 5 exp

PE
Enoxaparin 1mg/kg SC (LMWH)
Heparin 80U/kg bolus then 18U/kg/hr
Alteplase 10mg IV push, then 90mg over 2hr
If arrest: Alteplase 50mg IV bolus x 2 q15min

Sarah Foohey. Updated Sept 2021

CHAPTER 44
ACTION ITEMS

THE FOLLOWING action items can help you to prescribe medications safely:

- Prescribing medication requires assessment of **patient** factors, **disease** factors, and **medication** factors.
- Make note of **high-risk background problems** like CKD, cirrhosis, pregnancy, and advanced age that will influence your medication management plan.
- Review every patient's chart for their **home medications** and clarify that nothing is left off the list. If so, update the EMR to ensure no medication **interactions** are missed.
- For every unfamiliar diagnosis, **use a reliable reference** like UpToDate to find the first-line therapy, lab testing required for monitoring, and contraindications.
- Internalize the **"higher-risk medications list."** Whenever you consider prescribing one of these, double-check if a safer alternative exists, ask for guidance, use shared decision-making, and counsel your patients on when to stop taking them.
- Get your **pharmacist's** number on speed dial and don't hold back asking them questions.
- The best choice for **pain** management largely depends on the **patient's characteristics**. Be careful with elderly patients and those with chronic diseases like CKD. Use a pain control "ladder," starting with the safest options before escalating.
- **Nausea** is often safely treated with ondansetron but **beware of the patients at risk for long QT** (e.g., hereditary, those taking

other QT-prolonging medications, or suspected electrolyte disturbance). Most nausea medications prolong the QT.

- Have a **quick reference for medication dosing in emergencies**, even if you don't work in the ED.

Here are some **high-yield questions** to ask co-workers related to this section:

- What are the most commonly prescribed medications in our specialty?
- Of these medications, do any have serious risks to the point you avoid them when possible?
- What kinds of prescribing mistakes have you seen new grads making?

PART EIGHT
HOW TO COMMUNICATE AND DOCUMENT EFFECTIVELY

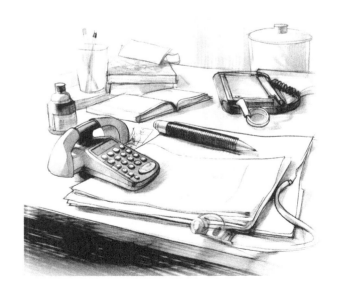

COMMUNICATION TREPIDATION

I'll never forget the story of my friend calling a consultation a few months into practice. Her experience up to that point was that specialists were short-tempered and rude, especially to new graduates. As a result, she was always nervous when making these calls.

One day she encountered a specialist who took her by surprise — they were warm and friendly. She connected so well with them that she accidentally ended the call with *"love you, bye"* as if speaking to a family member. She slammed the phone down, face beet red, and thought, "What have I done?!"

I felt the same anxieties before presenting or consulting as a new graduate. Interacting with so many strong personalities in medicine is daunting.

Patient presentations in phone consults are also an area ripe for pitfalls, especially for new graduates who think they must immediately accept whatever advice the physician specialists share. Unfortunately, getting bad advice from consultants is common for a variety of reasons. They aren't examining the patient or seeing the whole clinical picture. Furthermore, many are exhausted after taking night calls and understandably try to push back whenever possible for a better work-life balance. Regardless of the reason, bad consultant advice can result in bad outcomes, and you should do what you can to mitigate these situations.

Experienced clinicians know that the **quality of advice you get from these encounters reflects the quality of information *you provide to the consultant.*** Your consultants are incredibly busy. If you feed them a disorganized presentation without specifying your concerns, you set the entire team up to fail.

Some people are naturally good communicators who don't have to dedicate time to honing this skill, but *many* others are not. I certainly wasn't, and it's okay if you aren't either. I'll share the frameworks to use until it becomes second nature.

In the following chapters, we will review the following:

- How can you become a pro at calling consults?
- How can you best deal with bad advice?
- What strategies will help you communicate in a way that is rapport-building with patients?

- How can you document efficiently and defensively?

CHAPTER 45
ADVANCED STRATEGIES FOR CALLING CONSULTATIONS

During my first year out of school, of all my responsibilities, I found that calling consults was *the* most anxiety-provoking experience. My attending would tell me to call a consult for a given specialty, but I often didn't quite understand why and didn't know how to present a case efficiently. As a result, I was frequently yelled at by impatient consultants or admitters. I had no book to guide me and had to learn by trial and error.

This experience leads to my first advice: **grow a thick skin** and **don't take it personally**. The following guidance will help immensely but will not eliminate all negative encounters. The person holding the consult pager can sometimes be paged every few minutes while covering a service with more than fifty patients. If these consultants yell at you, chalk it up to a "systems problem."

COMMUNICATING IN CONSULTATION

Over the years, I've fine-tuned a framework that I use to present consults and admissions, and I haven't had a consultant angry at my presentation in a long time.

The process begins even before you send the page with a crucial pause for reflection: Do I **truly understand** the clinical situation, **the reason/question/request** behind the consult, and **the expected outcome?** Let's break these down one by one.

When you are new and haven't encountered a given clinical situation, **ask your attending before sending the page**, "Can you help me clarify our question or request, and why we can't act on our own? I want to be prepared when calling this consult."

You can't stop there. You need to reflect on **the consultant's potential responses** and **what you believe is the best option** for the patient. If the consultant gives you advice that is the *opposite* of what you anticipated, you should be ready to respond. More on this in a bit.

Now to the next step. Before you send the page, **put yourself in the consultant's shoes and consider what information they might need to answer your question.** Frequently, we forget to do certain parts of the H&P on the first pass because we aren't thinking from the consultant's perspective. They often want to know which specialist saw the patient last, the procedure/surgery details, catheterization reports, etc.

On my website, I have shared a list of **specialty-specific "vital signs"** that consultants always request. Some of these things might not be as relevant to you, but you'll be a pro if you have answers ready.

Here is an example of **"Nephrology vital signs"** you'd want to look up before calling a nephrology consult:

- Baseline eGFR and creatinine versus current?
- If on hemodialysis (HD): What days of the week? When was the last session? Did they complete a full session or not?
- Do they make any urine or not?
- Potassium (K) and bicarb levels.
- Is the patient volume overloaded centrally (lungs) or peripherally?
- Are any of the *"AEIOUs of emergent dialysis"* present? (e.g., **acidosis** with a pH <7.1, **electrolyte** problems like hyperkalemia >6.5, **intoxications** with dialyzable drugs like aspirin, **overloaded volume** like pulmonary edema, and **uremia complications** like encephalopathy or pericarditis.

―――――

Having done all the necessary prep work, you can send the page to your consultant. Next step: how do you present the patient's case efficiently and clearly? I use a condensed presentation roughly following the **ISBAR format** (Introduce, Situation one-liner, Background, Assessment, Recommendations):

You: "Hello, this is John, ER PA." (Introduce yourself.)

Consulting MD: "Hi, this is Dr. Jones, orthopedics, returning a page."
(Write down their name immediately — you must document this information.)

You: "We have a patient in Room 5, Ms. Rogers, with a hip fracture. We'd like to admit her and have your team consult. Would you like the MRN or the story?"
(Immediately state a one-liner summary to provide a frame of reference: basic patient info—the main problem—the specific request for them.)

Consulting MD: "Go ahead and tell me the story."

You: "She is a 65-year-old with a mechanical fall, landing on her right hip. She presented shortened and externally rotated, with X-rays confirming a displaced femoral neck fracture. She is neurovascularly intact. No other active medical problems, and she has been NPO since this AM. What else would you like to know?"
(Provide a **brief** summary of the clinical picture and workup results, share your working diagnosis, your question for them, and end by asking if they have clarifying questions)

Consulting MD: "That all sounds good. Admit her to medicine, and I'll add her to our list. Thanks."

CONTINGENCY PLANNING

The above example would be an easy consult to call because there is only one way to manage this situation (admission and surgery). The outcome should always be what you expect. However, many consults or admits are not so straightforward. The advice you get for patients in gray zones could be all over the map.

You should decide ahead of time what you think is in the patient's best interest. Discuss this **contingency plan** with your attending *before* sending the page if you anticipate a challenging conversation.

Ask your attending, **"If the consultant says to [admit and they'll see** the patient], great! If they say [they don't need to see the patient and we should discharge them to follow up], do we think that is safe?"

Coming to a conclusion ahead of time is important. If you determine the patient truly needs something, you can prepare your response to bad advice. That being said, you can't hound your consultants on every case. Pick and choose the battles to fight when necessary for a good health outcome.

DIALOGUE ACROSS DIFFERENCES

If you decide ahead of time that the patient needs a certain management plan, and the consultant recommends the opposite, how should you deal with this scenario? After all, you are a brand new APP standing up to an experienced physician specialist.

First, you must be clear with your consultant by **stating that you expected a different outcome**. They can't read your mind. You should then seek to understand whether the disconnect stems from a disagreement on the **diagnosis** or the **management.**

Consider a patient in the ED who we are concerned is developing a deep space hand infection that we think requires admission. We call hand surgery, who says the patient can go home with oral antibiotics. You might respond, "I hear what you are saying, but we feel that the patient needs to be admitted because we believe this is a case of flexor tenosynovitis (FTS). To clarify, was your understanding that we were dealing with FTS, or did you believe we are dealing with something else?"

- Potential consultant response #1: **"Oh, I didn't think we were dealing with [this diagnosis FTS] because there isn't a fever or a WBC elevation."** You would then respond by clarifying the point of confusion: "That is true, but on exam they have all of the Kanavel's signs, which has a high predictive value for FTS regardless of the lab results." They often concede and agree with the plan once we clarify our concerns.
- Potential consultant response #2: **"We agree on the diagnosis, but in my experience, most still do fine with oral antibiotics. I don't think they need surgery at this point."**

In the second case, with a disagreement on management, try to find that meet-in-the-middle option both parties can accept. Here is how I'd respond: "Of course I would defer to your expertise on the need for surgery or not. How about this — we will admit the patient to medicine and start them on IV antibiotics. If they improve with this, then your team can sign off. But if they worsen, can your team reassess the need for surgery?" Ninety-five percent of the time, the consultant will accept a middle-ground solution. If not, you may need to escalate to your attending or another supervisor.

―――

If you find that there is friction with your patient presentations to your attending, consider applying this framework to those situations as well. Before you present to them, reflect on what you think should be done and how you'd respond in a non-confrontational way if your attending recommends the opposite.

With time and practice, the approach in this chapter will soon become second nature and you'll enjoy calling consults. I certainly have come to love them. Through consultations, I've developed relationships with colleagues across every specialty. Each call serves a practical purpose and an opportunity to learn something new.

CHAPTER 46

BUILD RAPPORT WITH GOOD PATIENT COMMUNICATION

GOOD COMMUNICATION IS crucial for building rapport with patients, making accurate diagnoses, and ensuring patients follow your treatment plans. It will lead to happier patients and lower-stress interactions for you.

Setting a good first impression is vital. You don't want to do what one of my co-interns did. He entered the exam room and noted his patient (a woman in her thirties) and their older guest who had long hair. He said hello to the patient while gesturing towards the guest, "Did you bring your mother with you today?" The patient looked mortified and responded, "No! That is my husband!"

Upon closer inspection, he confirmed it wasn't an older woman but a middle-aged man with long hair. My friend learned a valuable lesson that he would not soon forget: Never assume who patients' guests are.

If communication doesn't come naturally to you like my friend above, don't worry. You can use the following scripting to set you up for success. Here's how I do it:

As soon as I enter the room, I say, **"Thank you for your patience."** After all, there is always a wait where I work.

I introduce myself and greet everyone in the room. If you see a guest, ask, "So, who did you bring with you today?" **Body language** is everything — I try to be open and warm. I avoid looking stressed or rushed.

I **sit on a chair by the bedside**, getting to their level. Best practice suggests staying off the computer, but I don't like to take charting home. I use the computer but maintain eye contact while typing.

Early in the case, I **ask about their concerns and their goals for coming**. This is the most important step to make your patients happy. They need to know that their goals and your goals align. You will undoubtedly hear patients say, "I went to another doctor, and they didn't do anything for me," yet when you review their chart, you see that they had ample testing and treatment ordered. That doctor likely failed to align goals at this step in the encounter.

After finishing my H&P, I **tell them my plan**. I am clear on what I order and how long it will take to get results. As I finish telling them the plan, I double-check that it addresses all of their goals for coming.

Under-promise and over-deliver on the time frame. If it takes an average of one hour to get test results back, say, "It can sometimes take up to two hours to get test results back, but we will try to expedite things for you." That way, they won't be upset if I sidetracked and it takes two hours.

As I walk out of the room, I find patients appreciate it when I do something simple like **turn down the fluorescent lights** and say, **"Please let us know if you need anything."**

For those who work in primary care who want to develop healthy long-term relationships with their patients, consider the following advice:

- Ask about their life, job, and hobbies — and **add a sticky note** to their chart. Sticky notes pop up each time you open their chart, so you can ask them about their favorite subjects when they return.
- **Get to know them as a person** beyond their medical history, by asking questions like, "What's your story? What brought you out this way? Did you catch the game last night? What's your favorite restaurant around where you live?"

COMMUNICATING UNCERTAINTY

A graduating student once asked me, "How should I communicate with patients when I don't know what is going on with them? I don't want to sound like an idiot!"

This is an excellent question. In these situations, we must walk the fine line between acknowledging we aren't sure and not conveying incompetence.

Consider these strategies:

- Demonstrate that you understand their **concerns**: "I'm also worried about your symptoms and we need to get to the bottom of it."
- **Be honest with them**: "I have an idea of what could be happening, but I'm not 100% sure. Sometimes the puzzle pieces don't fit neatly together and it can be challenging to sort out."
- Tell them your plan: "I want to get **a second opinion** with Dr. Jones before we proceed. We will work together to figure out the next steps." Patients love getting second opinions!
- Provide **reassurance** that you will do everything possible to give them excellent care.

TIME MANAGEMENT WITH "CHATTY PATIENTS"

New Grad APP: "So, Ms. Johnson, the intake note says you have a sore throat. When did that start?"

Chatty 60-year-old patient: "Well, you see, when I was seven years old, I fell off a horse and bruised my ribs like I had never experienced before. The horse was beautiful though, eight hands tall… [Unhelpful rambling ensues]."

Outpatient providers might only get fifteen minutes per visit, and the inpatient clinician might be juggling ten patients at a time. We all struggle with talkative patients who can't stay on-task.

There are various strategies to stay efficient. The book *Communication Rx* by Calvin Chou and Laura Cooley shares helpful advice —

- **Compassionate interruption to redirect the conversation**: "[Patient's name], I don't mean to interrupt you, but I want to ensure we have time for your exam. Can I ask you a few quick questions about your throat?"
- **Make a list with plans to address things later**: "What is everything you were hoping to address today?" Let them share their entire list, write it down, then follow with, "Great! Today we have time to address your chief complaint, and for the rest, we can schedule a follow-up appointment."
- **Summarize the visit to signal the end of the appointment**: "So, today we did an exam and ordered some diagnostic tests. You will start taking this medication and physical therapy. I'll message you with the test results in a few days. Let's follow up in two weeks to address the rest of your problems. If that all sounds good to you, I can walk you over now to the schedulers."
- **Have a backup plan if the above doesn't work**: I tell my support staff to knock and say there is a call for me if I am stuck in a room for more than thirty minutes. I very rarely have to use this, but with some particularly chatty patients, it can be a huge relief!

———

During your next shift, pay attention to your patients' body language as you speak with them. Do they appear receptive and understanding? Or do they seem unhappy and disengaged? If the latter rings true, consider checking out the above book, *Communication RX*. Authored by the Academy of Communication in Healthcare, the book draws from their extensive experience training healthcare workers to adopt effective communication skills.

CHAPTER 47

WRITING A PROFESSIONAL MEDICAL NOTE

"I am a PA student about to graduate. A common struggle I hear from new grads is staying late to finish notes. I've seen many preceptors have handy shortcuts that let them finish a note in less than five minutes. I have no idea how to make these shortcuts and would love tips on documenting efficiently."

THE LAST CHAPTER on communication involves charting. The medical record is your way of sharing what you think is happening and your management plan.

While I had opportunities to write notes in PA school, some rotations only allowed me to write the H&P and a "student's attempt" at the MDM. When I started my first job, it felt like the first time I was writing a complete note from start to finish. Writing down medical decision-making was a point of anxiety for me. Most new graduates express the same frustrations and questions:

- What is the purpose of a medical note?
- What should be included in each section of the note?
- Where can I find examples of notes to understand the format better?

This chapter addresses these questions and provides an overview of the components common across specialties.

The modern-day medical note serves three purposes:

- **Continuity of care**: We share the patient's clinical picture (symptoms, signs, test results), our assessment of what is going on, and our plan for them.
- **Defensibility:** Our note should demonstrate adherence to the standard of care in case of adverse outcomes and lawsuits. This involves things like documenting a DDx. In addition to saying what you think *is* going on, it is equally important to say what you feel is *not* going on. More on this below.
- **Billing:** Our note must capture the case's complexity to meet billing and coding needs.

NOTE CONTENTS

To start, the HPI section should generally include the **story** that the patient describes to you. This is written in medical terminology based on **our impression** of what they describe. A classic example is the parents who say their child is "lethargic," but when you look up, you see a child running around the room coloring on the walls. Lethargy is a medical term ("*A morbid condition of deep and lasting drowsiness that can only be aroused temporarily and with difficulty*"[1]) that the family might not appreciate. In this case, the family is describing relative fatigue, not frank lethargy.

The HPI also contains pertinent negatives related to whatever DDx you're considering. For a patient who presents with chest pain, you might write:

"59-year-old male with a PMH of HTN, HLD, presenting with acute onset of chest pain while at rest 5 hours prior to arrival. He describes a constant, pressure-like chest pain with radiation to the L arm.

He denies any leg pain or swelling, history of DVT/PE, recent surgery, or immobilization [PE DDx relevant negative ROS], [Aortic dissection relevant negative ROS], nor [Further DDx specific questions]."

---

1. "Lethargy | Definition & Symptoms | Britannica," February 10, 2023. https://www.britannica.com/science/lethargy.

Generally, the most important and challenging part for new learners is the Assessment/Plan/Medical Decision Making (MDM) section. An example note and a common outline of the MDM section might look like this:

[Summary Statement]

"60-year-old male with a PMH of ERSD presented with fatigue, nausea, and vomiting s/p missing three dialysis sessions. Pt presented hemodynamically stable and well-appearing overall. Workup notes several problems:

[Problem list and plan]

#hyperkalemia to 6.6. Mild T wave peaking. Treating with calcium, insulin, glucose, albuterol with resolution of EKG changes. Nephrology consulted and is arranging dialysis now.

#metabolic acidosis, anion gap elevation, we suspect it is related to renal failure and uremia. Bicarb is only mildly low at 17. Getting dialysis today. Nephrology reported we could hold on the bicarb gtt.

#mild pulmonary edema. O2 okay and pt. comfortable. Dialysis should correct.

[Risk management considerations]

We have also considered a broad DDx including but not limited to: ACS, doubtful with no chest pain, non-ischemic EKG, and troponin is baseline. Abdominal pathology, unlikely with benign abdominal exam and normal labs. Intracranial pathology, doubtful with no headache or trauma. Other emergent pathology is also less likely given that patient reports these symptoms are the same as prior epps of missing dialysis.

[for patients being discharged — include time and action-specific follow-up recommendations and return precautions]

HOW TO DOCUMENT YOUR DDX

You won't have time to write a long DDx for every patient. I recommend focusing your documentation solely on the lines of the DDx that have the following characteristics:

- The most likely condition, and your supporting evidence.
- The most dangerous condition(s), and why you don't think they're present.
- The conditions that **won't** be definitively ruled in or out with your testing.

Most clinicians consider it **unnecessary to document conditions that will be definitively ruled in or out with testing**. Suppose you have a patient with RUQ abdominal pain. Sure, they might have acute hepatitis, but there's not much value in documenting that possibility on a DDT when you'll know for sure after the LFT panel results.

Instead, **focus your DDx documentation on what you won't be testing for**. Explain why you don't appreciate red flags for appendicitis and thus don't think it's necessary to get a CT scan.

LEVEL UP YOUR DISCHARGE INSTRUCTIONS

In our M&M committee, one recurring theme is poor discharge instructions and how they increase our liability. The days of writing a simple "follow up as needed" and expecting patients to recall everything discussed verbally are over. Instead, provide them with specific time frames and action steps for follow-up.

A better discharge instruction template might look like this. Be sure to customize it for each patient:

"Thank you for visiting [location] today. Our assessment suggests that you most likely have [insert diagnosis]. We recommend starting [treatment X] and following up with [clinician Y] within [Z days].

Please remember that the diagnosis provided is our current impression, but we cannot be certain. You must [return or go to the ED] if your symptoms change or worsen, if you experience new symptoms, or if you notice [insert recommended return precaution signs and symptoms].

Additionally, our testing identified some abnormalities [insert incidental findings] that may not be related to your current symptoms but still require [follow-up plan]."

IMPROVE YOUR CHARTING EFFICIENCY

New grads frequently lament their charting inefficiency and must stay hours late catching up on notes. Ask your coworkers for their **templates and macros**. Most groups will have one "computer guru" who has done the leg work and shares their work with everyone else. There are great templates and macros for acute care at **ERnotes.net.**[2]

One pearl that I found particularly helpful was to **create pre-completed note templates as I studied the approach to chief complaints**. As I studied what history questions I was supposed to ask, exam maneuvers to perform, and testing to order for a given chief complaint, I created a pre-completed note that included this information.

For example, when I studied the approach to patients with ankle injuries, I learned the importance of asking for the mechanism of injury, whether they could bear weight and examining for a few key things (i.e., tenderness at the base of the foot, proximal fibula, and Achilles tendon region). I then created a note template for patients presenting with ankle injuries that included all of this information. The next time I saw a patient with an ankle injury, my note was 95% done with one click.

This method has three benefits:

- Pre-completed notes will **improve your charting efficiency**, helping you get home on time.
- You can open your note during your patient assessment to serve as a **real-time reminder of questions to ask and exams to do.**
- Studying the chief complaints and then immediately writing down the content into a document **helps to solidify the knowledge.**

2. ERNotes. "Home - ERNotes - ER Charting Made Simple." Accessed March 2, 2023. https://ernotes.net/.

REVIEW YOUR NOTE TEMPLATES FOR DEFENSIBILITY

For best practices in ensuring a defensible note, check out the resources provided by MedMalReviewer.com:

- *Documentation **Template***[3] - Provides an overview of the main points that should be covered in the MDM and goes into more detail than I covered above.
- *Documentation **Grading Rubric***[4] - Grades how defensible your care and documentation were via reviewing your note for specific criteria.

———

Documentation is an unavoidable reality of our jobs that even the most experienced practitioners lament. New grads often fall into the trap of over-documenting, recording every minute detail. As time goes by, you'll build a repertoire of pre-completed notes and begin trimming out the unnecessary parts of your documentation.

Your ultimate aim should be to finish all documentation during your shift, avoiding any carryover to your personal time. This goal is tough for many of us, but it can be done with practice and an eye for efficiency.

3. "Documentation Template." Accessed March 2, 2023. https://www.medmalreviewer.com/template/.
4. "Documentation Rubric." Accessed March 2, 2023. https://www.medmalreviewer.com/rubric/.

CHAPTER 48
ACTION ITEMS

THE FOLLOWING action items can help you to communicate and document effectively:

- Use **scripting** that sets a good first impression and addresses your patient's goals for coming.
- **Before sending any consult page, make sure that you know** (1) the reason for the consult, (2) the outcome you are expecting, (3) a contingency plan if you get the opposite advice
- Consider what information they'll need to answer your consult question — my website's **"Specialty Vital Signs"** list is a great place to start learning these.
- If you get bad advice, **let them know you didn't expect this advice, try to understand where the disconnect was** (diagnosis versus management) and **seek a middle ground** that everyone can accept.
- To learn charting at your first job, (1) ask for **templates** from your coworkers or use those shared online, (2) **get MRNs** from your shadow shifts and see what those templates look like filled out on real patients, (3) review your note template versus the **risk management rubric** to ensure it is protective.
- As you study the approach to your specialty's chief complaints, **create pre-completed notes** to serve as memory aids and efficiency boosters.

Here are some **high-yield questions** to ask co-workers related to this section:

- Which types of patients do you find the most challenging to interact with?
- What strategies have you found helpful in dealing with them?
- Which of our attendings are the biggest sticklers with patient presentations, and how do they prefer it?
- Are any of our consultant specialties known to give questionable advice?
- How would you advise dealing with these consultants?
- What changes did you make to your charting from when you started as a new grad?
- How are you able to finish charting during the shift so you don't have to take any home?

PART NINE
HOW TO RECOGNIZE AND MANAGE HIGH-RISK SITUATIONS

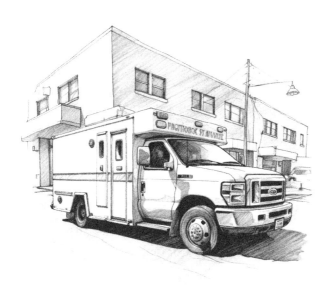

DEALING WITH UNCERTAINTY

"I graduated this year and have been practicing for a few months. I only feel confident in my diagnosis and treatment plan for about 40% of my patients. The rest, I think I know what to do, but I'm just not completely sure. What do you all do when in these situations?

Do you bother your attending physician when you feel uncertain? When is it safe to research online for the answer? When can I trust my gestalt?"

NEW GRAD EM PA, 2022

It will take years to feel confident in your diagnosis and treatment plans for most patients. For new grads, it is always better to err toward over-discussing cases with your attending. However, you'll soon learn that the decision to ask for help comes down to *the risk* of a dangerous condition or a bad outcome.

Healthy patients with benign complaints are at low risk — even if you aren't sure what is going on, it's probably okay to look things up on your own. However, patients with red flag features need more than educated guesses.

The book *Morbidity and Mortality* breaks down the clinical encounter into four factors that separate a low-risk from a high-risk case in a liability perspective.

The first factor is the **severity** of the illness, from mild to life-threatening. Second is the **obscurity** with which the disease presents, from very subtle to very obvious presentations. Third is the **provider's astuteness** during the encounter, including their assessment skills and medical knowledge. Fourth is the quality of the **patient-provider connection**. In other words, can they communicate effectively and build a good rapport with the patient in their care?

Combine all of those factors in a *negative* way, and you get a case of a lethal disease with a subtle presentation that meets an ill-prepared provider with a bad bedside manner. It's not going to end well.

On the other hand, many of these factors are within your control. Early on, prioritize learning about life-threatening or limb-threatening conditions, and focus on how they might present subtly or atypically. Improve your detection of red flags through study. Finally, have a good bedside manner and relationship with your patients. Do all these things and you will be well on your way to practicing medicine defensibly.

———

Assessing the risk of a patient encounter is a critical skill you must learn. In the next chapters, we will delve into this topic in greater depth:

- What *background* medical problems are high-risk? **(Online Bonus Chapter available with extra explanations)**
- What types of *patient presentations* are higher-risk than you might think? **(Online Bonus Chapter)**
- How important are *vital signs* in your risk assessment, and how should you react to abnormal vitals?
- What *cognitive errors* are new clinicians particularly prone to make in the face of red flags?
- What are the *risk-mitigation best practices*?
- What are the *most commonly missed diagnoses* that result in patient harm and malpractice, and how can I avoid missing them? **(Online Bonus Chapter)**
- *Case practice: Pattern recognition cases* for high-risk conditions in adults and pediatrics. **(Online Bonus Chapter)**

Due to the book's length constraints, I have moved a few topics from this section to **Online Bonus Chapters**, which are available for free on ClassroomToClinician.com under the "Resources" section. If the bolded topics interest you, please check them out on the website.

CHAPTER 49
THE RISK RADAR

How can we identify patients at risk of dangerous pathology and bad outcomes? General rules of thumb can sometimes give a rough estimate of any patient's risk. I trained with a hilarious emergency physician who taught the following:

The risk of serious pathology = The patient's **age** divided by the **number of complaints.**

Suppose you have a 25-year-old male with no PMHx who complains of difficulty sleeping, dry skin, itchy teeth, and four more complaints on the review of systems. He has had prior workups and specialist visits, all unrevealing. Even if you are uncertain about the cause of his symptoms or what to do for him, it is a low-risk situation and wouldn't warrant bothering your attending. Contrast that with the 80-year-old man who comes in with one complaint, "acute vertigo," and he has an 80% chance of something bad going on.

If only our jobs were as easy as plugging simple information into a risk calculator like this. In real life, you'll have to develop a radar that detects high-risk features in every part of the clinical assessment.

The prior chapters on clinical decision-making introduced this topic, and we will now narrow our focus on the highest-risk findings you may encounter. All of the following findings put your patient at significantly higher risk for deterioration than your average patient. Thus, make special note if your patient has any of these and be prepared to activate the risk-mitigation steps discussed in a few chapters.

PATIENT FACTORS

- End-stage organ dysfunction (e.g., advanced heart failure, ESRD, liver failure, etc.).
- Immunocompromised states (e.g., AIDS, poorly controlled DM).
- Significant cardiac disease, vascular disease (e.g., severe PAD), or critical aortic stenosis.
- Advanced lung disease (e.g., severe COPD).
- Patients with coagulopathies (e.g., factor V Leiden) or bleeding disorders (e.g., hemophilia).
- Myasthenia gravis.
- Late-term pregnancy and post-partum period.
- Metastatic cancer.
- Neutropenia.
- Pulmonary hypertension.
- Adrenal insufficiency.
- Organ transplant history.
- Roux-en-Y gastric bypass history.
- "Device patients" (e.g., LVAD, VP shunt, etc.).
- Homelessness.
- Intravenous or illicit drug use.
- Severe alcohol use disorder.

PRESENTATION FACTORS

- Red flag symptoms, which require dedicated study to learn (e.g., "the red flag approach to headache").
- Sudden onset symptoms (e.g., thunderclap headache or chest pain).
- Exertional worsening of symptoms or dyspnea.
- A sign or symptom that is progressively worsening over time.
- Systemic infectious symptoms without a clear viral source like an upper respiratory infection.
- Physical exam abnormalities related to the cardiac, vascular, or neurological exam.

- Any functional impairment (e.g., "I can't walk anymore," or, "My mother is not making any sense when she talks").
- Abnormal vital signs (discussed next chapter).
- Patients who *look* seriously ill (e.g., pale, diaphoretic, toxic appearance).
- Bounceback patients (covered in online bonus chapter).
- Against medical advice discharge (covered in online bonus chapter).

CRITICAL VALUE TEST RESULTS

- Test results marked with two exclamation points "!!" on the EMR indicate a critical value.
- Other red flag lab results, as discussed in the prior chapter.
- Critical imaging findings include anything mentioning a vascular blockage, ischemia, necrosis, gas/air in an area it isn't supposed to be, or the need for urgent specialist consultation.

CLINICIAN FACTORS

- Is your "spidey sense" telling you something bad is happening with the patient?
- Is your nurse telling you they're worried about the patient?
- If so, listen!

The lists above are not all-inclusive but should give you a sense of the types of things to hone in on during your assessments. If you identify *any* one of these red flags, you should classify the patient as higher risk. This might seem like overkill, and it will be in many cases. For example, patients with one abnormal vital sign often turn out fine.

While experienced clinicians might know when it is safe to disregard a red flag, it takes years to know when it's safe to do so. It's prudent for new grads to have a low threshold to put the patient into a high-risk category. The next steps, which we will review in an upcoming chapter, mainly involve slowing down and being thorough. In other words, there is no harm and a lot of potential benefits with this approach.

Next, let's review the nuance of vital sign abnormalities in risk assessment.

CHAPTER 50
THE APPROACH TO ABNORMAL VITAL SIGNS

YOUR RED FLAG radar should always be attuned to abnormal vital signs. Whereas the patient interview gives us an abundance of subjective data, vital signs provide objective information that directly reflects the physiologic state of the body.

What's more, abnormal vital signs are one of the few things studies have repeatedly found to correlate with worse outcomes. One study found that ED patients with one abnormal vital sign at discharge had twice the rate of bad outcomes, and patients with two or more had three times the rate.[1] Tachycardia and hypotension had the greatest risk of poor outcomes.

As the saying goes, **vital signs are vital.** Yet, they are so frequently abnormal and many new grads aren't sure how to react. It's helpful to have a stepwise approach to these situations. Here's how experienced clinicians do it —

---

(1) __Identify the abnormal vital sign:__ This first step needs to be called out because some new clinicians don't have the habit of reviewing vital signs for every patient. After identifying an abnormal vital sign, **compare it to the patient's prior vital signs** to if it's their baseline. Many patients will have baseline systolic blood pressures in the 90s or heart rates in the 40s.

---

1. Gabayan GZ, Gould MK, Weiss RE, Derose SF, Chiu VY, Sarkisian CA. Emergency Department Vital Signs and Outcomes After Discharge. Acad Emerg Med. 2017 Jul;24(7):846-854. doi: 10.1111/acem.13194. PMID: 28375565; PMCID: PMC5935002.

(2) **Try to correct it:** You can use measures like antipyretics if the patient is febrile with tachycardia, or fluids if the patient is dehydrated. If they are bradycardic, does it correct when the patient walks around? If the abnormal vital sign is easily corrected, this is considered more reassuring. If not, we consider "persistently abnormal vital signs" more of a red flag.

(3) **Assess whether or not they are symptomatic:** The clinical picture trumps all. It is concerning if they have red flag signs or symptoms plus abnormal vital signs. However, if they are completely asymptomatic, this is less concerning. For example, marathon runners often have benign sinus bradycardia, but they are asymptomatic.

(4) **Try to identify the underlying cause:** Ensure you've thoroughly addressed their chief complaint and reviewed all test results to find a cause. If none is apparent, reflect on whether the vital signs can lead you to the answer. Emergency medical conditions are essentially derangements of vital functions, and the patterns can give clues to the problem.

Low blood pressure plus tachycardia suggests a shock state, which can be further narrowed with the pulse pressure. A wide pulse pressure suggests a distributive shock state like sepsis. A narrow pulse pressure suggests a low output shock state like cardiogenic shock.

High blood pressure plus tachycardia may suggest a sympathetic surge state, like methamphetamine use or alcohol withdrawal. A high respiratory rate (hyperventilation) with normal oxygen saturation might suggest acidemia like DKA. Hypoxia most often localizes the problem to the lungs (e.g., COPD) or cardiovasculature (e.g., heart failure with pulmonary edema, pulmonary embolism, or shunt state).

Your physical exam can assess a few other key physiological indicators to help narrow the cause. My favorite quick bedside exams for these patients are JVD and the extremities' temperature. An elevated JVP helps indicate there is heart failure from a cardiogenic or obstructive problem. Extremity temperature (i.e., warm extremities with brisk cap refill versus cool and mottled extremities) can also help differentiate between the major categories of shock.

Check out the fantastic figure from the Internet Book of Critical Care at the end of this chapter to learn more about how these can be used in conjunction with bedside ultrasound to substantially narrow the DDx.[2]

(5) **Escalate care for higher-risk vitals:** Not all abnormal vital signs share the same weight. My rule of thumb is to be most worried when there's significant **tachypnea (24+), tachycardia (110+), hypoxia (<94%), or hypotension (SBP<100)**. I admit these patients even if I still haven't found a diagnosis. New grads are encouraged to consult their attending. The other vital sign abnormalities like fever and elevated blood pressure might not be as predictive of sinister pathology in an otherwise benign clinical picture.

All abnormal vital signs must be addressed in some way. Most of the time, "addressing it" is as simple as rechecking their heart rate after resting for ten minutes, or reviewing the prior visits and confirming their blood pressure is at baseline. We then put a documentation blurb to that effect. However, having this practice will help improve your detection of sinister conditions. I regularly pick up patients with subtle pathology because of an unexplained and uncorrectable abnormal vital sign.

The teaching point: Addressing abnormal vital signs in practice *and documentation* is an essential risk-mitigation strategy.

---

2. https://emcrit.org/ibcc/shock/

bedside approach to undifferentiated shock/hypotension

	IVC or Jugular vein size	Lung POCUS	Significant pericardial effusion	RV dilation	LVEF	Mitral or aortic regurg?	Cardiac Output
Distributive shock - Septic shock* - Anaphylaxis* - Adrenal crisis◻, Thyroid storm - Post-cardiac arrest SIRS - Pancreatitis, Hepatic failure - Neurogenic (trauma, spinal anesth) - Vasodilatory medications	↓↓ or normal	Normal (or focal abnormality from pneumonia)	-	-	nl / ↑	-	**High output:** - Warm extremities. - Low diastolic Bp. - Wide pulse pressure. - May be febrile. - May look toxic. - Capillary refill is variable.
Hypovolemic shock - Vomiting, diarrhea, overdiuresis - Hemorrhage (GI, peritoneal, RP) **Abdominal compartm. syndrome**	↓↓↓	Normal	-	-	nl / ↑	-	**Low output** - Cool extremities. - Diastolic Bp may be normal.
RV failure - PE, - Decompensated chronic PH - RV myocardial infarction	↑↑	Normal	-	**+**	nl / ↑	-	- Narrow pulse pressure. - Delayed capillary refill.
Tamponade	↑	Normal	**+**	-	nl / ↑	-	
Tension pneumothorax	↑	No slide on affected hemithorax	-	-	nl / ↑		
AutoPEEP / high airway pressure - Asthma > COPD > ARDS - Exacerbated by hypovolemia - Dx based on history, vent waves	nl/↑	Normal	-	**+/-**	nl / ↑	-	
LV failure - MI - Myocarditis, postpartum CM - Takotsubo cardiomyopathy - Beta-blocker overdose	nl/↑	B-lines everywhere	-	**+/-**	**↓↓**	**+/-**	

CHAPTER 51
COGNITIVE ERRORS AND RISK MITIGATION BEST PRACTICES

CLINICIANS REACT to red flags in many different ways. In this chapter, we will study the **types of mistakes** new clinicians are prone to making. We will share the **situations** that most strongly predispose us to errors. We will then review the **general risk-mitigation best practices** to apply to all patients. The last chapter will conclude with a **targeted approach** to the highest-risk patients you face.

THE TOP 5 COGNITIVE ERRORS IN CLINICAL MEDICINE

Ultimately, errors come from a failure to identify high-risk features or a failure to respond to them appropriately. But *why* does this happen? Let's review the most common cognitive errors that can affect your decision-making as a new clinician:

- **Anchoring bias:** When you latch onto early features of a case and ignore later data that suggest an alternative diagnosis. For example, the patient with dyspnea and cough in whom you anchor on the possibility of pneumonia despite later noting bilateral leg edema suggesting congestive heart failure.
- **Availability bias:** Judging things as more likely when they're fresh in your mind. After seeing a grand round's case of a patient with Guillan Barre syndrome, you suddenly find this diagnosis popping into your head when your next patient complains of weakness. While good to consider, it should be lower on the DDx given how rare the condition is.

- **Blind obedience:** Immediately accepting the recommendations of an expert without independently considering whether the recommendations are sound. This is an incredibly common occurrence with new grad APPs, who don't think it's their place to refute a specialist or their attending's recommendations. Specialists and attendings can be wrong too, so be prepared with the scripting from the communication chapters to address your concerns in a non-confrontational way.
- **Confirmation bias:** Seeking data that supports your hypothesis while ignoring data contradicting it. In the above patient case of pneumonia versus congestive heart failure, the novice clinician might specifically ask whether the patient has a productive cough and confirm they must have pneumonia. If they had kept an open mind and probed further, they'd have noticed the subtle detail that the productive cough only occurs when the patient lays flat.
- **Diagnosis momentum:** Once a patient is labeled with a diagnosis, it sticks in our minds and influences our interpretation of other data. Even a simple comment from a triage nurse, "Oh, it's just another cyclic vomiter," can impact how you subconsciously assess the patient. This ties in similarly with **Premature closure bias.**

These aren't hard concepts to grasp, but it can be challenging to recognize when they're happening to you. It's easier to recognize the *situations* these most commonly occur. When you find yourself in any of these situations, recognize that you're in a situation primed for error:

- **The bounceback patient who is worsening despite your treatment plan:** This is a classic setup for anchoring bias, diagnosis momentum, and premature closure bias. Force yourself to expand the DDx to consider alternatives.
- **The patient who was seen by another doctor and carries an "established diagnosis:"** Trust, but verify! Make sure you independently evaluate the patient and agree with their conclusion. The **patient handoff at shift change or transfers** holds the same risks.
- **The "frequent flyer" patient:** Like the boy who cried wolf, these patients may also develop serious pathology and shouldn't be

ignored. Go through the same systematic approach as any other patient and don't ignore red flags.

- **The "hard to deal with patient"**: This includes patients with psychosocial challenges like severe drug use or homelessness. Your support staff might roll their eyes when you say they need a workup. But if a workup is indicated, they deserve one just like anyone else.
- **The language barrier patient:** It can be tempting to let the patient's teenage child interpret for them on busy shifts, but don't cave in. Explain that a professional interpreter is essential.
- **The against medical advice (AMA) discharge**: You might think you're protected medicolegally if they went against your advice, but you'd be wrong. The rate of bad outcomes — and lawsuits — is higher in these patients. The online chapter shares how to approach these patients and document defensibly.
- **The last patient at the end of your shift**: You'll be tired and find yourself making medical decisions that you wouldn't have earlier, like skipping indicated testing. We have seen a number of quality cases occur in these situations. Resist the urge and follow your practice pattern regardless of how painful the late shifts can be.

If you find yourself in these situations, be sure to implement the strategies listed in the next chapter. My favorite experts who teach these topics are Drs. Greg Henry and Rick Bukata. They are both legends in emergency medicine and medical malpractice experts. They run a paid podcast called *Risk Management Monthly*, which delves into the core content of high-risk medicine. If you're interested in subscribing, I'd recommend checking out the oldest episodes just as much as the newest ones, as they are packed full of pearls and still very relevant to practice today.

They share two important pearls that every new graduate must know. **First, never alter a medical record after the case has ended if you later hear of a bad outcome**. Writing an updated MDM after you know the true diagnosis is a gift to the plaintiff's attorney and demonstrates that you've realized a mistake. If you must amend something, whatever you write must be the truth, time-stamped, and clearly labeled as an addendum.

Second, if you don't put a note in the chart, your malpractice insurance won't cover you! There are a variety of situations this can come up:

- A patient calls the nursing line asking for medical advice, and you do the nursing staff a favor by answering their questions.
- You are sitting behind the front desk when the nurse asks you to eyeball a patient she is worried about before sending them back to the waiting room.
- Your medical assistant asks you to look in their ears and throat to see why they're having pain.

Malpractice insurance carriers are paid for each patient encounter generated by the patient's chart. If you didn't leave a note, they were not paid and are not obligated to cover you should a bad outcome result.

The teaching point: Do what you can to avoid cognitive errors, document every piece of medical advice you give, and don't give any advice for free, or you'll be the one to pay.

CHAPTER 52
MANAGING RISK WITH BEST PRACTICES

My GOOD FRIEND LUKE JOHNSON, PA-C, accurately summarized the challenges of these chapters:

"Real-life patient scenarios aren't at all like those on board exams. Our tests share a straightforward presentation with clear right and wrong answers. In practice, most patients have an unclear presentation that doesn't fit any one disease. You're left considering four different management options, all of which might be wrong. If there's anything I've learned, it's the importance of getting comfortable with uncertainty."

Uncertainty will be high as a new grad and gradually improve, but never fully disappear. You're now equipped with a red flag radar and some general best practices for every patient encounter. Once you've identified a high-risk patient, what then is the best way to deal with them?

Step one: *Slow down.* Our work demands us to work quickly for most patients we see. However, for the subset of high-risk patients, you must slow down and pay special attention to each step of the patient encounter.

Step two: *Go over and above to develop a good rapport with the patient and family.* This can't be said enough. Tell them why you are concerned and that you'll take great care of them.

Step three: *Investigate the red flags further.* Do a thorough history and physical to identify any other red flags. Ask yourself what disease you think is present and what else could it be. Generate a DDx and compare the patient's symptoms to each line of the DDx to see if there is a match. Ask yourself if any finding doesn't fit with your suspected diagnosis.

Step four: *Come up with your own preliminary plan.* Even if you have no idea what to do, it's okay to make your best guess. Pretend you are on your own, what do you think would be the best way to manage this patient? These moments of critical thinking will help you grow significantly in your first year.

Step five: *Involve your attending physician and compare their plan with yours.* Then, make it happen and deliver great patient care.

RISK MITIGATION BEST PRACTICES

While risk mitigation strategies are most essential in high-risk patients, they are **great habits to apply to all patients.** They decrease medicolegal risk and are simply good patient care. This is an expanded list of best practices to consider. You'll notice some recurring themes from throughout the book.

Communication:

- Use the communication chapter techniques to **cultivate a good rapport** with your patients. Happy patients are more likely to follow treatment plans and less likely to pursue litigation.
- Speak to your patients in **lay terms** so they understand the gravity of the situation. Avoid using medical terminology.
- **Review nursing and other provider notes** and document any discrepancies with your evaluation. For example, triage notes or referral orders might include a red flag like "sudden onset

headache" — it's our job to follow up on these and clarify in our documentation if it's a concern.

- In your discharge instructions, highlight the importance of **strict return precautions** for any new or worsening symptoms. This is especially true for those with negative test results.
- Provide **time-specific** and **action-specific discharge instructions.**
- Give **well-organized patient presentations** to consultants with a clear question or request for them. Think critically about each case and **be prepared to manage poor consultant advice.**

Clinical evaluation and decision making:

- Use a **systematic approach** in your patient assessment to note **red flags** and develop a plan to address each one. Document their presence or absence in your note.
- Address **all abnormal vital signs.**
- Pay particular attention to your **vascular exam** and **exams of function** (e.g., neurological, tendon/ROM) and always work up abnormalities with them.
- **Consider and document a brief DDx** for straightforward cases and **a more thorough DDx** for higher-risk cases. Consider dangerous possibilities first.
- Review your clinical data prior to disposition to consider whether anything suggests *against* your working diagnosis.
- Implement **cognitive forcing strategies** into your practice. For example, "Every time I have a bounceback patient, I will consult my attending."
- Consider general **admission criteria** regardless of patient presentation.
- Only **prescribe medications** when they are actually indicated. Tell the patient about **risks** like sedation so they know to avoid driving. Be careful prescribing **high-risk medications** and take the follow-up steps if they are required.

Documentation:

- **Finish your charts as soon as you can.** If you later note your patient decompensated, do not edit your chart retroactively, as this can be tracked and presumed a cover-up for fault.
- Be careful with completely **generic pre-completed notes or macros**, as plaintiff lawyers can accuse it of not being accurate. Try adding something unique to that patient's presentation in each chart, like, "Pleasant and conversational man in the exam room with his daughter."
- Document your **medical decision-making.** Include your targeted DDx and considerations for serious pathology.
- Discuss and document all required aspects for **informed consent, shared decision-making,** and **leaving against medical advice (AMA).** These need to be documented in a specific way to be protective and are discussed further in the online bonus chapters.
- Review your note template versus the **defensibility grading rubric.**

Your ability to detect high-risk situations will improve as you gain experience. If you want to study this area for faster growth, consider the following three strategies.

First, join your local peer review or morbidity and mortality (M&M) committee. These groups review high-risk cases, dissect the documentation, and discuss ways to prevent these bad outcomes in the future. They are excellent learning opportunities, and our new graduates who attend universally say they grow from the experience.

Second, set up a system to periodically review your high-risk patients. Use your EMR to generate reports on your patients who bounced back or were admitted after your care. You can also manually add challenging patients to a reminder list. The system will prompt you later to review what happened with the patient. You can also call to see how they are doing. Getting feedback on your care is very helpful to grow as a clinician.

Third, explore the best medico-legal resources to deepen your understanding —

- *Risk Management Monthly Podcast*: A fantastic paid podcast by the best in the field, as discussed earlier.

- *Bouncebacks!*: An interactive book series sharing real patient cases that resulted in poor outcomes.
- *Malpractice Insights Newsletter*: A free email sharing closed claim cases with lessons learned.
- *Expert Witness Newsletter*: A paid email newsletter with more frequency than others.
- *Morbidity and Mortality Rounds in EM*: An older book with patient cases and take-away teaching points.
- *Avoiding common errors in the emergency department*: A great book by Dr. Amal Mattu summarizing classic pitfalls in EM.

Although studying high-risk situations may initially seem stressful, mastering them can reduce your anxiety and help you become a more confident practitioner.

CHAPTER 53
ACTION ITEMS

THE FOLLOWING action items can help decrease your risk of missing serious conditions and your liability:

- **Know when to reach out for help.** This is a function of the situation's risk.
- **Many factors reliably increase the risk**, like high-risk background medical issues (PMH, surgeries, and meds), unique patient populations (the bounceback or AMA patient), or those with red flags.
- **Study the cognitive errors** we are all prone to, **the situations** they most commonly manifest, and **the strategies** to prevent them.
- **Focus your studies** on the classic *and atypical* **presentations of dangerous conditions.** Most misses are from atypical presentations of common pathologies like heart attacks and strokes.
- **Address abnormal vital signs** in your management and charting.
- **Implement best practices** like good discharge and follow-up instructions. Include a plan for all incidental findings.

Here are some **high-yield questions** to ask co-workers related to this section:

- Are there patient presentations that our specialty considers particularly high-risk?
- What are the most commonly litigated diagnoses in our specialty?
- How do you deal with these high-risk situations?
- What are the most common reasons new grads end up on quality review?
- How did you learn to avoid these pitfalls?

PART TEN
HOW TO LEARN THE CLINICAL MEDICINE OF YOUR SPECIALTY

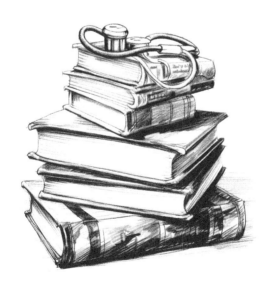

STUDYING CLINICAL MEDICINE FOR THE LONG-HAUL

"Studying in grad school felt like drinking from a firehose, yet everyone says we've only scratched the surface of what we will need to know. That's kind of terrifying. I think what would help me is some blueprint of the content I haven't learned yet and advice for how to learn it all."

GRADUATING FNP, 2024

Until this point of the book, my primary goal has been to equip you with strategies (e.g., SPIT DDx) and tools (e.g., M.D.Calc) to assist you while caring for patients on shift. I chose this approach because it can have the biggest impact in the shortest time. However, these will only get you so far. You still must study medicine to become the expert that clinical practice requires.

However, learning medicine is a massive endeavor. You will only fully appreciate this after several years of practice. I recently looked at my notes from PA school on a Powerpoint set for electrolyte abnormalities. At the time, it felt like an overwhelming amount of information. Now, I know that each bullet point of the Powerpoint could have an hour lecture in and of itself. I didn't truly understand hyponatremia until I heard it explained by experts in three different specialties.

Takeaway #1: Learning clinical medicine is hard.

Some will look up at the mountain of a challenge ahead of them, get overwhelmed, and not have the will to continue studying. Others will try to sprint up the mountain, studying hours each day to the point of burnout a few months in.

Takeaway #2: Learning clinical medicine is a marathon, not a sprint.

You'll need to devise a study plan to chip away at this challenge over several years. Research suggests a great approach is "tiny habits" with easy-to-achieve daily routines.

. . .

n the following chapters, I will share an approach to studying with the end goal of becoming an expert. We will discuss the following key ideas —

- **Prioritize what content to learn first**: the approach to the chief complaints of your specialty is the highest yield.
- **Create a study plan:** This plan must be easy to accomplish even on your busiest days.
- **Use the best sources**: This section's final chapters divide the best resources by specialty.

CHAPTER 54
THE HIGHEST-YIELD CONTENT

THE FIRST AREA TO focus on is the approach to your specialty's chief complaints or clinical problems. For example, assessing chest pain in emergency medicine or hyponatremia in internal medicine. These are the fundamentals of any specialty and should be studied first.

Action item: Search online for the "**top 20 most common chief complaints and problems of [your specialty]**." Begin working from most common to least common. Use the highest quality sources to learn this content.

Below is the general content to be learned within the context of a chief complaint. **Prioritize learning the bolded content first**, as the others can be more easily looked up during your shift.

- **Differential diagnosis (DDx).**
- **Essential history** questions, focusing on **red flags associated with that complaint.**
- **Physical exam** to perform.
- **Standard order set** to workup this chief complaint. Understand each order set's rationale, limitations, and common variations.
- Targeted treatment once the definitive diagnosis is established.
- When does this issue require emergent consultation with a specialist, non-emergent follow-up with the specialist, or primary care follow-up?

- Disposition considerations, such as admission or discharge criteria.

CHIEF COMPLAINT-SPECIFIC RED FLAGS

Studying the red flags unique to each chief complaint is essential for every new grad. For better or worse, many patients come to us with a myriad of symptoms, negative testing, and we can't ever find the exact cause of their symptoms. We can then say, "No red flags for serious conditions are present. Whatever else it might be, we have time to sort it out."

This line of thinking is built into the approach for many chief complaints. There is the "red flag approach to headache, back pain, rashes, and more." In these approaches, the emphasis is not on pinning the patient into a *single diagnosis* but rather on ensuring no sinister *category* of diseases is present. After ruling out that category, you can start nonspecific treatment for the basket of "everything else."

However, you can't stop at simply identifying red flags. You need to study *why* those H&P features are considered red flags in the first place. What conditions should they make you consider? This type of content is harder to look up on shift and dedicated study is essential.

I didn't quite grasp this concept when I started practicing. I once had a patient who came in with back pain. I learned the red flag approach to back pain, and the patient mentioned having incontinence on the ROS. I patted myself on the back for recognizing a red flag and immediately went to my attending to present the case.

My attending responded calmly, "Okay, your back pain patient has incontinence, got it. Tell me more. What kind of incontinence? Is it new or old? Does she have a mechanism by which she could get cauda equina syndrome (like cancer, IVDU, injury, known spinal stenosis, etc.)? Does she have any objective findings or deficits on exam, like sensory, motor, or deep tendon reflex changes? Does she have saddle anesthesia or diminished rectal tone? Can she walk? What was her post-void residual bladder scan?"

My attending didn't actually ask that many questions, but the point is that I didn't know the answer to any of those things. You'll be ahead of the average new grad if you learn the *next* steps after identifying the red flag.

In the above case, the patient might have clarified, "Oh, I have always had this incontinence, it happens when I sneeze, and there is nothing new today." If she screened negative for all those other clarifying H&P items, it would be perfectly reasonable to discharge her.

CHAPTER 55
TINY HABITS FOR LIFELONG LEARNING

CREATING a consistent study routine is the next piece of the puzzle. The easier it is to complete, even on busy days, the better. Try to integrate studying into your daily activities and make it a habit.

One approach is to bundle studying with another established routine. Identify triggers for your study habit: "Every time I get in my car, I will open my podcast app to find a new episode." You'll have to figure out what works best for you, but in this chapter, I'll share some ideas to help you brainstorm.

These **five habits** have grown my medical knowledge more than anything else and I still do them to this day:

1. On shift, **I write down knowledge gaps** as they arise on my phone's app. The app acts as a storage ground for easy-access questions for #2 below.
2. During quieter moments at work, **I ask my senior colleagues** for their thoughts on the questions from my phone. I ask the same questions to *multiple clinicians* to get a sense of practice variation and the rationale behind each approach.
3. During commutes, **I listen to medical podcasts,** selecting episodes related to knowledge gaps. Actively seeking out information significantly enhances long-term retention.
4. I keep a **specialty textbook on my bedside table** and read a few

pages every night before bed. This habit not only reinforces learning but also doubles as a sleep aid.

5. I have a **recurring calendar reminder** each January to look up the best conferences of the year and ask off work for them.

Reflect on your learning style and consider what kind of system would be sustainable and effective. By employing this approach, you can maximize learning every day without the need to carve out large chunks of time outside of work.

CHAPTER 56
ACUTE CARE TRANSITION PLAN

WE ARE APPROACHING the end of the book and will now begin to tie everything together. This chapter shares a game plan for those starting in emergency medicine, urgent care, and other specialties treating patients with acute complaints. Use this as a blueprint with the best resources to organize your studies.

———

Begin by studying the approach to acute care's most common chief complaints. Here is the list in descending order of frequency:

- Traumatic and orthopedic injuries (e.g., falls, MVC, etc)
- Fever, cough, sore throat, and other infectious complaints
- Back pain
- Abdominal pain, vomiting, or diarrhea
- Urinary symptoms
- Pelvic complaints (e.g., discharge, pain, STD exposure)
- Rash
- Headache
- Eye pain or redness
- Dental pain
- Chest pain
- Dyspnea
- Dizziness or vertigo
- Altered mental status

- Weakness
- Hypotension

EM:Rap's C3 content is the highest quality resource for learning how to approach these complaints. Academic Life in EM shares an **intern survival guide**[1] that reviews other core content and landmark studies. The **EMRA Chief Complaint Pocket Guide** and **Wikem.org** can be used on shift for quick reference. They also share the **order sets** you need to work up your patients.

As you see patients, you will apply what you've learned to order the right tests. Once you get these test results back, use **Wikem to reference specific disease management and disposition guidance.** It tends to be more acute care specific than UpToDate.

If you work in fast track or urgent care, **don't drop your guard for simple chief complaints or low acuity triages.** Seek out the pertinent red flags in each case. Check out the famous "fast track disasters" thread by Eric Holden PA, DHSc (@EMEDPA) that brings this teaching point to life.[2]

When juggling multiple patients, **prioritize care with this hierarchy**: (1) sick patients, (2) patients ready for disposition, and (3) new patients. Keep your patient list on the tracker board sorted by longest to shortest "length of stay," and collaborate with nurses to facilitate dispositions.

For urgent care providers, review FP Notebook, WikEM, and UpToDate **to determine if your patient needs to be sent to the ED.**

Once you've mastered the chief complaint approaches, focus on the rest of the EM core content blueprint[3] shared by NCCPA. Here are the top resources to help you study these topics:

- **EM:Rap and UC:Rap** - Comprehensive paid resources covering a wide range of emergency medicine topics through podcasts and articles. This is the best one-stop shop for everything you need to learn acute care.
- **EM:Crit** - A paid resource focusing on high-acuity and advanced procedures in emergency medicine.

1. RDMS, Jeffrey Shih, MD. "ALiEM's Greatest Hits for Interns: A Curated Collection of High-Yield Topics." *ALiEM* (blog), July 21, 2017. https://www.aliem.com/greatest-hits-interns-curated-high-yield-topics/.
2. Physician Assistant Forum. "'it's Probably Nothing'-Fast Track Disasters," May 30, 2005. https://www.physicianassistantforum.com/topic/30-its-probably-nothing-fast-track-disasters/.
3. https://www.nccpa.net/wp-content/uploads/2021/06/EMContentBlueprint.pdf

- **EBMedicine** - Evidence-based updates to emergency medicine core content through articles and reviews.
- **WikEM** - A quick reference website for emergency medicine topics and guidelines.
- **EM:Clerkship** - A free website and podcast providing basic core content and real-life case examples in emergency medicine.
- **Rosen's** Emergency Medicine and **Tintinalli's** Emergency Medicine - Comprehensive textbooks covering all aspects of emergency medicine.
- **Emergency Medicine Cases** - A free website and podcast discussing various emergency medicine topics and cases.
- **Pediatric Emergency Playbook** - A podcast and website focusing on pediatric emergency medicine.
- **ECGs for the Emergency Physician** - A book covering ECG interpretation for emergency medicine providers.
- **Dr. Smith's EKG Blog** - A free website dedicated to EKG interpretation and case discussions.
- **EMRA Antibiotic Guide** - A reference guide for antibiotic selection in emergency medicine.
- **Avoiding Common Errors in the Emergency Department** - A book that addresses common pitfalls and mistakes in emergency medicine.
- **CHOP Pathways** - Guidelines and algorithms for pediatric complaints in emergency medicine.
- **Bouncebacks!** Book series - A series of books discussing challenging cases and lessons learned in emergency medicine.
- **First10 EM and Foohey's Figures** - A free website covering various emergency medicine topics, including case discussions and educational resources.
- **ACEP Clinical Practice Guidelines** - Guidelines from the American College of Emergency Physicians to ensure evidence-based, standardized care in emergency medicine.

Here are some great **conferences** for new graduates:

- EM Bootcamp
- SEMPA 360 Conference
- Urgent Care Association Annual Convention & Expo
- Emergency Nurses Association (ENA) Annual Conference

Embrace your new role in acute care and use these resources to guide your learning journey!

CHAPTER 57
PRIMARY CARE TRANSITION PLAN

THIS CHAPTER WILL OFFER practical guidance and resources for those who will work in primary care. The wide breadth of this specialty presents an immense challenge, but let's break it down into manageable steps.

Start by studying the approach to the chief complaints of family medicine, from most common to least common:

- **Hypertension**: diagnosis, the workup for secondary causes when indicated, monitoring, and management.
- **Diabetes** diagnosis and management.
- **Hyperlipidemia**.
- **Preventative care**: Immunizations, health screenings, and counseling on lifestyle modifications for disease prevention.
- **Asthma** and **COPD**.
- **Allergies**.
- **Infections**: Skin infections, ear infections, upper and lower respiratory infections, and STIs.
- **Gastrointestinal complaints**: Acid reflux, irritable bowel syndrome, constipation, and diarrhea.
- **Anxiety** and **depression**: screening, diagnosis, and therapy options.
- **Musculoskeletal pain:** Back pain, joint pain, acute and chronic.
- **Headaches** and **migraines**.
- **Skin conditions:** Assessment and treatment of rashes, acne, eczema, and dermatitis.
- **Thyroid** disorders.

- **Urinary tract infections.**
- **Women's health:** Menstrual disorders, contraception, menopause, screening like HPV / Paps, and more.
- **Pediatric care:** Routine well-child exams, immunizations, and management of common childhood illnesses.
- **Geriatric care:** Management of chronic conditions, medication adjustments, and addressing age-related concerns in older adults.
- **Weight management.**
- **Sleep disorders.**

Preview your schedule for the coming day to see their complaints. The **best resources to study the approach to chief complaints** are the American Academy of Family Practice (AAFP) practice articles and UpToDate. Search for Curbsiders and Clinical Problem Solvers podcast episodes to listen to them apply this knowledge as they work through real patient cases.

Pocket Primary Care and 5-Minute Consult are print options for **quick references** while at work. Family Practice Notebook is an excellent online reference. They provide order sets to help you work up patients.

Improve efficiency by saving custom order sets for common complaints like yearly physicals and vaccines. Maximize the use of your support staff. Have them manage as much of your inbox as possible. **Icontraception** offers guidance for the safest contraception options.

As you see patients, you will apply what you've learned to put in the right orders for them. Once you get these test results back, use FP Notebook to reference **disease-specific management and disposition guidance** if you have ruled in a diagnosis.

The following resources can help **determine if your patient needs to be sent to the ED**:

- FP Notebook.
- UpToDate.
- WikEM.

Once you have learned the chief complaint approaches, switch your focus to studying the rest of the **FM core content blueprint** shared by NCCPA[1]. Here are the highest-quality resources to learn this content —

---

1. https://www.theabfm.org/sites/default/files/2019-02/FMCOneDayExamBlueprint.pdf

- The Curbsiders.
- AFP Podcast.
- CoreIM.
- UpToDate.
- Prescriber's Letter.
- Huppert's Notes Textbook.
- The Internal Medicine Pocket Medicine Book.
- Guide to Most Common Internal Medicine Workups.
- 5 Min Pediatric Consult.
- The Harriet Lane Handbook.
- Fitzpatrick's Dermatology.

Here are some CME conferences for new graduates:

- American Academy of Family Physicians (AAFP) Family Medicine Experience (FMX).
- American College of Physicians (ACP) Internal Medicine Meeting.
- Primary Care Network (PCN) Destinations Conference.
- National Association of Pediatric Nurse Practitioners (NAPNAP) Annual Conference.
- American Association of Nurse Practitioners (AANP) National Conference.

WHEN SHOULD I REFER TO SPECIALISTS?

When I was researching the content for this book, I found many new family medicine APPs were insecure about the decision of when to refer to a specialist. For example, which diabetic patients need a referral to endocrinology, and which should be managed by family medicine?

No single resource lists all indications for referrals because it is location-dependent. I'd first try references like FP Notebook, UpToDate, American Academy of Family Practice (AAFP), American College of Physicians (ACP), and the Family Physician Journal for guidance on when to refer and how you can start initial treatment. At times the respective specialty society (e.g., American Academy of Neurology) might also have indications for referral on their website or guideline documents.

You can also ask whether the local specialists offer **"tele-consults"** or phone calls to determine whether a referral is warranted and if they want you to send any panels or start any preliminary treatment in the interim.

Last, the **Curbsiders** website and podcast focus heavily on outpatient internal medicine and have many great resources for practical clinical questions like when to refer.[2]

Ultimately, you should seek help if you don't feel comfortable managing your patient and aren't sure where to go next. Ask your senior colleagues or attending for input.

---

2. https://thecurbsiders.com/episode-list

CHAPTER 58
THE BEST RESOURCES FOR OTHER SPECIALTIES

OVER THE YEARS, I have bookmarked what I consider the "best of the best" lectures and content sources. Whenever I hear others sharing similar praise in other specialties, I add their recommendations. This chapter will share that list with you. If you don't feel confident in your knowledge of the topics from this list, these resources would be a fantastic place to start your studies.

CRITICAL CARE:

- Dr. Reuben Strayer's **"Emergency Thinking"** lecture (Youtube video) - How the real-world approach to sick patients differs from what is taught in school.
- Curbsiders **"Rapid Response Series:" Acute hypoxia podcast episode**.
- **EM:Crit** (paid website and podcast) - Emergency medicine and critical care resources, including podcasts, blog posts, and educational content.
- **Internet Book of Critical Care** (free website) - Housed on the EM:Crit site, a fantastic reference for core content.
- **Critical Care Scenarios** (free podcast) - Podcast run by APPs in critical care and the most common scenarios they face.
- **OnePager ICU** (free website) - Fantastic summary infographics on ICU-relevant topics.

- **Deranged Physiology** - Excellent website to understand the 'why' behind challenging topics.
- **Critical Care Reviews** - A resource offering reviews and summaries of the latest research and developments in critical care.
- **SMACC Podcast** - A podcast focusing on critical care, emergency medicine, and prehospital care.
- **PulmPeeps -** A podcast that discusses various pulmonary and critical care medicine topics.

CARDIOLOGY

- **Kittleson Rules Heart Failure lecture**, Curbsiders Epp 230, one of their most watched episodes.
- **Emergency arrhythmias 101 lecture** - Dr. Laurel Brown Louisville Lectures (Youtube).
- **Atrial fibrillation - Curbsiders Epp 159** - Excellent episode discussing the diagnosis and management of atrial fibrillation.
- **Stress testing 5 Pearls** on CoreIM Podcast - Best summary of the core concepts related to cardiac stress testing.
- **Approach to EKGs ST elevation and wide complex,** ERcast Amal Mattu - A discussion on how to approach ST elevation and wide complex EKGs.
- **Life in the Fast Lane** (free website) - Content across many topics, most famous for their EKG content.
- **The Cardiology Show** - A podcast that covers cardiology-related topics, interviews with experts, and discussions on current events in cardiovascular medicine.
- **CardioNerds** - A podcast by cardiology fellows that discusses various cardiology topics and offers case-based learning.
- **American College of Cardiology (ACC)** website - Visit the ACC website for clinical resources, guidelines, and educational materials related to cardiology. You can also subscribe to the Journal of the American College of Cardiology (JACC).
- **Circulation** - A prestigious cardiology journal focusing on original research and reviews in cardiovascular science and practice.

HOSPITAL MEDICINE

- **Clinical Problem Solvers** (free and paid material, website and podcast) - The best source for improving diagnostic skills and approaching undifferentiated patients, with great diagnostic schemas.
- **CoreIM Podcast** (free podcast and website) - The highest quality podcasts and content I've ever heard on bread and butter IM core content. Highly recommended!
- **Curbsiders** (free podcast and website) - THE internal medicine podcast with expert interviews sharing practice-changing knowledge. Start by listening to the "Reboot" episodes, the most popular episodes on their platform.
- **Louisville Lectures** (free on Youtube) - Internal medicine lectures for daily didactics are recorded and uploaded for all to watch, covering a wide range of topics.
- **Febrile, A Cultured Podcast** (free podcast) - Infectious disease fellow brings practice cases and experts to reason through them out loud.
- **MedCram** (e.g., Acute Kidney Injury Explained Clearly) - A series of medical video lectures covering various topics, including acute kidney injury.
- **The Curious Clinicians** - A podcast exploring medicine's fascinating and less-known aspects, focusing on internal medicine, pathophysiology, and clinical reasoning.
- **Run the List Podcast** - A case-based podcast that evaluates and manages common medical problems encountered in the hospital setting.
- **Internal Medicine Survival Guides** (multiple found freely online) - Collection of guides and manuals focusing on practical management of internal and hospital medicine problems.

NEUROLOGY

- **Approach to dizziness:** Curbsiders Epp 49 with Dr. David Newman (neurologist and lead researcher on vertigo), Dr. Peter John's Youtube videos, and EM:Crit podcast episode 316 Vertigo.
- **Stroke and TIA deconstructed** - Curbsiders Epp 164 - A

comprehensive discussion on diagnosing and managing stroke and transient ischemic attack.

- **Cervical artery dissection** - Rutgers Neurology video on Youtube - An educational video on the diagnosis and management of cervical artery dissection.
- **Cerebral venous thrombosis** - EMCrit Epp 304 CVT - A podcast episode discussing the evaluation and treatment of cerebral venous thrombosis.
- **Neurology Exam Prep Podcast** - A podcast covering various topics in neurology, useful for exam preparation and clinical practice.
- **Lange Clinical Neurology and Neuroanatomy**: A Localization-Based Approach by Dr. Aaron Berkowitz - A comprehensive neuroanatomy and clinical neurology resource. Listen to Dr. Berkowitz on the CP Solvers Neuro VMR podcast.
- **American Academy of Neurology (AAN)** - Visit the AAN website for clinical resources, guidelines, and educational materials related to neurology.

PSYCHIATRY

- **PsychDB** (website) - A daily-use resource with diagnostic criteria and first-line medications for various psychiatric disorders. Highly recommended by PHMNPs.
- **The Carlat Psychiatry Podcast** (free podcast) — Hosted by a psychiatrist and a PMHNP, this podcast offers consistently excellent content.
- **The Carlat Report newsletters** (General Psych, Addiction Treatment Report, Hospital Psychiatry, Geriatric Psychiatry, Child Psych) - Highly recommended newsletters providing valuable updates and information in various psychiatric specialties.
- **The Psychiatry & Psychotherapy Podcast** - A podcast that covers various psychiatry topics, interviews with experts, and discussions on current events in psychiatric medicine.
- **Simple and Practical Psychiatry** (website) - A resource with concise, practical information on various topics in psychiatry.
- **Psychopharm Institute** - A resource focused on the psychopharmacology of psychiatric disorders.

- **Stahl's Essential Psychopharmacotherapy** - A comprehensive textbook covering the principles and practice of psychopharmacology.
- **American Psychiatric Association (APA)** website - Visit the APA website for clinical resources, guidelines, and educational materials related to psychiatry. They also have an annual conference.

GENERAL AND TRAUMA SURGERY

- **Behind the Knife Podcast** - A podcast discussing various topics in general surgery, including case reviews and interviews with experts.
- **Surgery 101 Podcast** - A podcast series focused on essential topics in general surgery.
- **Touch Surgery -** Surgical Videos (App) - A mobile app offering a library of surgical videos and simulations for educational purposes.
- **Dr. Pestana's Surgery Notes** - Top 180 Vignettes for the Surgical Wards (Book) - A collection of high-yield vignettes covering various surgical topics.
- **Surgery - A Case-Based Clinical Review** (Book) - A comprehensive book that presents various surgical cases and reviews the relevant clinical information.
- **"Essentials of General Surgery"** by Peter F. Lawrence - A comprehensive textbook covering the core principles of general surgery, excellent for both new and experienced clinicians.
- **American College of Surgeons (ACS)** website - Visit the ACS website for clinical resources, guidelines, and educational materials related to surgery.
- **"ATLS: Advanced Trauma Life Support"** by the American College of Surgeons - A widely used resource for trauma care that provides a systematic approach to the initial assessment and management of injured patients.
- **"The Trauma Manual:** Trauma and Acute Care Surgery" by Andrew B. Peitzman, Michael Rhodes, C. William Schwab, Donald M. Yealy, and Timothy C. Fabian - A practical, concise guide to the management of trauma patients, covering a wide range of topics related to trauma surgery and critical care.

- **Eastern Association for the Surgery of Trauma (EAST)** website - Visit the EAST website for clinical resources, guidelines, and educational materials related to trauma surgery.
- **The Trauma Professional's Blog** - A blog and podcast by Dr. Michael McGonigal that covers trauma-related topics and case discussions.
- **Trauma ICU Rounds -** A podcast series discussing various topics in trauma surgery and intensive care management.

ORTHOPEDIC SURGERY

- **OrthoBullets** - A comprehensive online resource with articles, videos, and quizzes on various orthopedic topics.
- **Nailed It Podcast** - A podcast covering various orthopedic surgery topics, including case discussions and expert interviews.
- **The Handbook of Fractures** textbook by Drs. Koval and Zuckerman - A comprehensive guide to diagnosing and managing fractures.
- **McRae's Orthopedic Trauma** - A textbook focusing on managing orthopedic trauma injuries.
- **Practical Office Orthopedics** - A resource that covers common orthopedic issues encountered in outpatient settings.
- **Handbook of Splinting and Casting** - A guide to the proper techniques and materials for splinting and casting.
- **Netter's Concise Orthopaedic Anatomy textbook** - A visual resource that presents orthopedic anatomy using detailed illustrations.
- **Hoppenfeld Surgical Exposure** - A textbook that covers surgical approaches and techniques in orthopedic surgery.
- **Orthopedic Galaxy Conference**: an AAPA CME Course - A continuing medical education course for orthopedic providers.

Is there a specific lecture you've heard that is the "best in class?" If so, please send it to me, and I'll add it to future versions of the book. Contact me at StanglMedical1 at Gmail.com

CHAPTER 59
ACTION ITEMS

THE FOLLOWING action items can help you learn the clinical medicine of your specialty:

- Develop a **personalized study routine** that is easy to continue for years.
- As you work, **write down the gaps in your knowledge** as they come up.
- Study the topic using the **highest quality resources.**
- As you study their resources, prioritize retention on the approach to the **chief complaint**, identifying **red flags**, and avoiding **iatrogenic harm.**

Here are some **high-yield questions** to ask co-workers related to this section:

- What resources have you found the most helpful to learn the clinical medicine of our specialty?
- What do you think are the best conferences for our specialty?

THE MEGA SUMMARY: FROM CLASSROOM TO CLINICIAN

We've reached the end of the guidebook, and it's time for the mega summary. Everything started with you, the intrepid new graduate APP. I remember the new grad reality —I've been there and the memories remain fresh in my mind. We are excited, scared, and overwhelmed as we start our careers. We have a never-ending to-do list, which this book has likely added to.

Let's take a step back and remember why this book exists in the first place. Practicing medicine as a new grad is **hard**. I hope this book has enabled you to break down this complex challenge into manageable pieces. Let's distill all the action items into one chapter.

To practice medicine safely and confidently as a new grad, you'll need to do the following...

1. Find a safety net job: This is the most important step toward your goal of safe practice. Unfortunately, finding a job with great support and a gradual ramp-up is difficult. How can you make it happen?

- **Cast a medium-sized net** with two to three specialties in a broad geographic zone.
- **Cast your net in the right places.** Start with your network and local websites before the generic job boards.
- **Leverage automated casting technology** by setting up job alerts and website change detectors to be the first one to apply.
- **Craft a stellar application** that stands out from the crowd.

- **Practice the best answers** to the questions they'll ask you during interviews.
- Take the **list of questions to uncover red flags** with you to the interview.
- When faced with multiple job offers, **prioritize support and mentorship.**
- When faced with no suitable offers, **consider a residency program.**

---

2. Overcome counterproductive emotions like imposter syndrome: When you start your first job, *expect* to feel low confidence. We all experience these feelings, so remember you are not alone. The ideal mindset for the new graduate is a humble acknowledgment of your clinical limitations paired with enthusiasm and determination to grow. Create a plan to practice medicine safely that you are happy with, and trust the process. It still won't be easy, and you'll encounter many low points. Remember your motivations, adopt a growth mindset, and take it one step at a time. You'll notice that things will get better with each passing week.

---

3. Ramp up quickly with the 80/20 rule: Your first month's focus should be learning the 20% of medicine you'll use 80% of the time. This includes the most practical aspects of the job, like working up the most common problems of your specialty:

- Search online for your specialty's *top twenty patient presentations* and *survival guides.*
- Research and ask coworkers for *ordersets, algorithms*, and *references* to aid in working up these patients (e.g., FP notebook, Wikem.org, Pointofcaremedicine.com, and Uptodate.com).
- If you prefer print resources, buy a high-quality *on-shift reference.* EMRA's Basics of EM Pocketbook, Guide to Most Common Internal Medicine Workups, and Pocket Primary Care are great options.

Important note: Make a DDx and a problem list for each patient to fill in the gaps that ordersets miss.

4. Level up your clinical problem-solving skills: The ordersets above are only a temporary solution until your assessment capabilities develop. What can you do to improve your evaluation skills?

- Use a systematic approach for every patient to avoid missing things.
- Use a prompt system like the one detailed (i.e., Background - Foreground - DDx - Testing - Treatment - Disposition) to help spur your memory during your evaluations.
- Interpret diagnostic test results accurately, using external references like schemas to aid you.
- Pause to review data, sort into signal vs noise, and make a problem list.
- Make a summary statement focusing on the strongest signals to guide the next steps.
- When tests come back negative, pause to consider whether tests with poor sensitivity might have missed anything on your DDx.
- Learn from the masters — Subscribe to RLR Clinical Problem Solvers to hear the best teachers in the business apply these concepts.
- Periodically review your challenging cases with a mentor.
- Practice your critical thinking skills with simulated cases.

---

5. Be a cautious prescriber: First, do no harm! The following action items will reduce your medication errors:

- Study the shortlist — your specialty's top twenty most commonly prescribed medications, focusing on potential harms.
- Download the best medication references (e.g., UpToDate, Epocrates, and FirstLine).
- Follow the "safe prescribing habits."
- Learn the list of high-risk medications, be careful when prescribing them, consider alternatives, and use shared decision-making with your patient.
- Double-check medication choices when prescribing to high-risk patient populations like those with chronic organ failure.

- Get your pharmacist's number on speed dial.

---

6. Know when to reach out for help: This is a function of the *risk of the patient encounter* – in the patient's background, presentation, or workup results. Develop your red flag radar for each section. Whenever you encounter a patient with a red flag in the background or foreground, categorize them as high-risk patients and proceed to risk mitigation steps.

Learn the most common new grad errors in the face of red flags. Study cognitive errors like anchoring bias and diagnosis momentum. Recognize when you are in situations where mistakes flourish, like in patients returning for failure to improve.

---

7. React appropriately when you encounter a high-risk patient: Slow down, spend extra time on your H&P, think critically, make a strong DDx, assess the possible causes, develop your action plan, and then ask your attending for help. Compare your plan to theirs to learn from each case.

The risk-mitigation best practices are general steps to take for every patient to improve their care. They include actions like giving good discharge instructions, addressing abnormal vitals, and writing a defensible chart.

You can improve the quality of your care by joining your local morbidity and mortality committee, periodically reviewing your high-risk patients with a mentor, and reading the best medico-legal books (e.g., The *Bouncebacks* series).

---

9. Communicate and document like a pro: Ask your coworkers for the level of detail your attendings and consultants will want in patient presentations. Review the "specialty vital signs list" to learn what specific information consultants want to hear in your reports.

Before calling specialist consults, make sure you know (1) the specific question/request for the consultant, (2) the answer you expect, and (3) a contingency plan if you get the opposite advice.

Ask your coworkers for charting templates or use the ones shared online. Compare them to the defensible charting rubric. As you study core content, make pre-completed notes for each chief complaint. This will help with your charting efficiency and help you recall important assessments when you perform your H&Ps.

———

10. Develop tiny habits that make lifelong learning easy: It will take several years to learn the clinical medicine of your specialty. Small chunks of "ninja studying" daily are more sustainable than the long study sessions you did in school.

You'll have to find the habits that work best for you, but consider starting with the following:

1. *Write down gaps in knowledge* in your phone as they arise on shift.
2. Fill in the knowledge gaps with *medical podcasts during commutes.* Use the highest-quality medical podcasts list.
3. During slower periods at work, *ask senior coworkers questions that remain on your list.* Ask multiple coworkers to get a feel for practice variation.
4. Set a recurring calendar reminder to schedule time off for a *high-quality CME conference* yearly.

———

FEEDBACK REQUEST

We are now nearing the end of the book, with just the conclusion and bonus sections on personal finance remaining. I would like to pause and ask for your feedback:

- **Do you feel the content has effectively addressed the book's goal?** (i.e., How to practice medicine safely and confidently as a new graduate)
- **Are there any questions or confusing areas arising from the content?**
- **Do you have any suggestions to improve the book further?**

I will use your feedback to improve the book for future readers. I'm also happy to answer any questions you may have. Please email me at StanglMedical1 at Gmail.com or message me via the contact section of my website ClassroomToClinician.com.

CONCLUSION

At the beginning of this book, we discussed the knowledge gap every new graduate faces. I hope this book has been your bridge, enabling you to stride across the turbulent waters of your first year in practice. With the foundations of safe practice firmly laid, you'll soon stand on the other side of the bridge with paths spreading in all directions. All the hard work will soon pay off, and life will only get better from here!

I want to thank you for reading the new grad guidebook. Please let me know if it helped you by emailing me or connecting with me via the contact page of my website, **ClassroomToClinician.com**.

If you believe in my mission of helping new graduates, you can support me in the following ways:

- **Leave a review** on Amazon via the link or QR code on the next page — it helps more than you realize!
- **Join the e-mail list** on my website or via the QR code on the next page to be notified about future content. I plan to share future free content with those on my email list.
- **Share the book's Amazon link** on social media.
- **Recommend the book** when you encounter students, new grads, or anyone who asks what to buy with their CME funds.

I wish each of you the best of luck in your journey. —JS

QR Code to leave Amazon review:
(http://www.amazon.com/review/create-review?&asin=B0CDJQND8V)

QR Code to join email list:
(ClassroomToClinician.com/Email-List)

Many of my beta readers requested a review of personal finance relevant to new PAs and NPs. I've included two bonus chapters in the appendix, coming up next.

APPENDIX: BONUS CHAPTER 1 — PERSONAL FINANCE FUNDAMENTALS

If you've made it this far in the book, you've likely got your first job as an APP with a big paycheck coming. How can you make the most of it? I studied personal finance for years after graduation. I'll share what I learned in this chapter.

Here are the basics of personal finance that every new graduate should understand:

1. Optimize your **income** and keep your **expenses** in check to generate a **monthly surplus.**
2. Use that surplus intelligently so your money **compounds in** *your* **favor.**
3. Purchase the critical personal finance adjuncts, such as **life** and **disability insurance,** to protect your growing nest egg.
4. Fine-tune your plan with **further study from the best sources.**

STEP 1: HOW TO OPTIMIZE YOUR INCOME AND EXPENSES

You have already taken steps to **negotiate for a higher salary.** How do you keep that hard-earned income in your pocket? If you have the means, a great first step is to max out your pre-tax 401(k). At an APP's income level, taking off the top $20,000 of your income by contributing it to your 401(k) pre-tax will immediately yield about **five thousand dollars per year** saved from your income that would otherwise have been taxed.

The beautiful thing about maxing out your 401(k) via payroll is that you won't even know what you're missing. You combat lifestyle inflation by taking money off the top for investment rather than for unnecessary expenses.

This leads us to the other side of the income coin: **Expenses**. Be mindful of your expenses when first starting. If you can continue living frugally for a few years with a few meaningful lifestyle upgrades, it will serve you well in the long term.

STEP 2: USE THE MONTHLY CASH SURPLUS WISELY

Everyone's financial situation is unique, but some commonly recommended flowcharts give you an idea of the options available with the surplus you are left with at the end of each month. My favorite flowchart can be found on the personal finance forum on Reddit:

https://www.reddit.com/r/personalfinance/wiki/commontopics

They recommend starting with a few key steps:

- Build an emergency fund.
- Max out your employer-sponsored match funds through a 401(k).
- Pay down high-interest debts.

If you still have some money left over after these steps, you are in a great place. Next, you can try to pay down student loans and consider contributing to a **Roth IRA**. You can do this via a **backdoor** Roth IRA if you exceed the income limit. Check out the White Coat Investor Backdoor Roth IRA blog post for step-by-step guidance.

You'll need to select how to invest the funds you've put into your 401(k) and Roth IRA. I am not a financial adviser, so I'll only explain the basics. Investments come in a few forms. There are **active investments** such as day trading, choosing an actively managed fund, and using a money or investment manager, to name a few. These generally have high fees and variable returns on your investment. There are also **passive investments** with low-cost index funds that tend to have minimal fees and will perform the same as the whole market you've selected.

Passive investing has been popular for decades, and I chose this route when comparing the two. My favorite book is J.L. Collins' *The Simple Path to Wealth*, which convinced me of the power of passive investing.

Practically speaking, I use **Boglehead's 3-Fund Portfolio** of index funds: One total US stock fund like VTSAX, one broad-based international stock fund like VTIAX, and one bond fund like VBTLX. Your age and risk profile will determine the breakdown percentage of stocks versus bonds, as detailed in the linked webpage.[1] I select funds like these in my 401(k), Roth IRA, and taxable brokerage accounts. I set up my accounts to **automatically invest a certain amount each month** from my payroll and bank account so that I don't need to put much time or energy into maintaining a solid financial plan.

STEP 3: OPTIMIZE YOUR PERSONAL FINANCE "ADJUNCTS"

Disability and life insurance go beyond earning, spending, and investing, so the next bonus chapter will cover them in detail. These are a critical part of your personal finance plan.

STEP 4: DETAILED SOURCES TO LEARN MORE

Of the many different personal finance resources I've read, the **financial independence, retire early (FIRE) movement** has provided the most practical advice. However, learning about the FIRE movement does not require you to retire early if you don't want to. The movement focuses on valuing free time more than money and optimizing personal finances to win back more time to do the things you love. They provide everyday people with actionable tips to accomplish these goals. If that sounds interesting, consider checking out the following resources:

- **ChooseFI** (Podcast/Website)
- **Madfientist** (Podcast/Website)
- **MrMoneyMustache** (Podcast/Website)
- **The Personal Finance Subreddit**
- **Bogleheads** Wiki and Forum
- **The Compound & Friends** (Podcast/Website)

Now that you have a good foundation, let's move to a more in-depth review of the personal finance adjuncts.

---

1. https://bogleheads.org/wiki/Three-fund_portfolio

APPENDIX: BONUS CHAPTER 2— PA & NP DISABILITY INSURANCE

While I had always enjoyed reading about personal finance and investing, the insurance domain had initially felt more complicated and out of reach. My initial reaction was to avoid insurance products altogether. Unfortunately, the reality is you cannot avoid insurance if you want a sound financial plan.

My research found that the educated financial and medical communities recommended **disability insurance** for healthcare workers, *even if they don't have dependents.*[1,2] This protects your most valuable asset, your income, essentially cementing a solid income for the rest of your life.

They also recommend **term life insurance** for those *with* families or dependents. Let's review some more rules of thumb…

A) PEOPLE AND PRODUCTS TO GENERALLY AVOID:

- **Brokers who are affiliated with only one company**, and therefore can't give you any real comparisons.
- **Whole life insurance.** This is considered a poor investment choice by many. I chose term life insurance, which meets my

1. Investor, The White Coat. "Understanding Disability Insurance for Doctors | White Coat Investor." The White Coat Investor - Investing & Personal Finance for Doctors, July 23, 2022. https://www.whitecoatinvestor.com/what-you-need-to-know-about-disability-insurance/.
2. "Disability Insurance for EM Physicians." Accessed July 27, 2023. https://www.emra.org/residents-fellows/financial-planning/disability-insurance.

family's needs and nothing more, and is the most affordable option.

- **"Any-occupation" disability insurance.** In this plan, if you have an injury that prevents you from working in medicine, the insurer can refuse your disability claim and say you can find a job in a different field.

B) BETTER ALTERNATIVES:

- Find an *independent* **insurance broker** to help you find term life and long-term disability insurance. They can plug your information into a system and provide quotes from multiple companies. If you can, meet with various brokers to see whom you'd prefer and ensure their quotes are fair. You will provide all your health, personal, and bank account data, so you want to find trustworthy people. I used the White Coat Investors website list and was very happy with the broker I chose.
- Select a broker who **works with APPs and our unique needs** for insurance. For healthcare providers, the gold standard is to get **own-occupation, specialty-specific long-term disability insurance.** With this coverage, if you lose the function of a hand and can't work in your specialty, you'd still be covered by the insurance plan. More on this below.

KEY ADVICE: APPLY EARLY

The White Coat Investor and many others highly recommend getting disability insurance as soon as possible for multiple reasons, so I'd encourage you to start this process now. The benefits of early application are two-fold. First, the younger you are, the more affordable the policy will be. The rate at which you sign up will be locked in for the rest of your career, so it benefits you financially to sign up early.

Second, you'll have fewer exclusions for pre-existing medical conditions. Most students put off going to the doctor for anything until they graduate, at which point they get health insurance and "catch up on their healthcare needs." If you wait to get disability insurance until after these visits, the insurance company will list every problem as an exclusion they won't cover. If you lock into an insurance plan before you have these problems, they'll all be covered conditions down the road.

PA/NP-SPECIFIC CONSIDERATIONS

As a PA trying to find *specialty-specific* own-occ coverage, I quickly discovered that this search gets muddy. PAs, at least, do not have specialties ingrained into our boards and licensing. Luckily, I found a broker who had experience with this situation, interacted extensively with the insurance companies on my behalf, and we did our best to make the case that my "profession" was an *emergency medicine* PA.

It was interesting diving into the fine print with him and seeing how important it was to choose the specific insurance company, as each company has unique phrasing in their policies that might support our goal or not. Passing the EM boards and getting a certificate of added qualifications (CAQ, the specialty boards for PAs) was another big step we took to this end. Ultimately, the specialty-specific occupation determination for an APP will come down to a case-by-case judgment if there is a claim. You can do many things to support your position, and your broker can help you form the foundation needed ahead of time.

I would encourage you to find a few agents to compare. In part of your comparison, consider trying my agent Pradeed Audho. He is very knowledgeable about the unique APP experience and is an independent insurance broker for disability and life insurance. His website is https://pkainsurance.com. I had a great experience working with him and would highly recommend him.

ACKNOWLEDGEMENTS

I want to sincerely thank the following individuals who provided significant feedback to help shape the book into what it is today:

- Jian Li Zheng
- Toni Nelson
- Gordon Stangl
- Jennifer Psujek, Editor
- Luke Johnson, PA-C
- Cody Balogh, PA-C
- Scott Kluth, NP
- Ashley Kneale, NP-S
- Kelcey Webster, PA-S

Made in the USA
Las Vegas, NV
22 September 2024

95665482R00193